Water Fasting

Water Fasting to Heal Your Body and Lose Weight Effectively

(Rapid Weight Loss, Revitalized Health and Body Cleansing Through Water Fasting)

Brian Madden

Published By **Daniel Kaplan**

Brian Madden

Water Fasting: Water Fasting to Heal Your Body and Lose Weight Effectively (Rapid Weight Loss, Revitalized Health and Body Cleansing Through Water Fasting)

ISBN 978-1-7386412-5-3

Legal & Disclaimer

The information contained in this book is not designed to replace or take the place of any form of medicine or professional medical advice. The information in this book has been provided for educational & entertainment purposes only.

The information contained in this book has been compiled from sources deemed reliable, and it is accurate to the best of the Author's knowledge; however, the Author cannot guarantee its accuracy and validity and cannot be held liable for any errors or omissions. Changes are periodically made to this book. You must consult your doctor or get professional medical advice before using any of the suggested remedies, techniques, or information in this book.

Upon using the information contained in this book, you agree to hold harmless the Author from and against any damages, costs, and expenses, including any legal fees potentially resulting from the application of any of the information provided by this guide. This disclaimer applies to any damages or injury caused by the use and application, whether directly or indirectly, of any advice or information presented, whether for breach of contract, tort, negligence, personal injury, criminal intent, or under any other cause of action.

You agree to accept all risks of using the information presented inside this book. You need to consult a professional medical practitioner in order to ensure you are both able and healthy enough to participate in this program.

Table Of Contents

Chapter 1: The Rich History Of Water Fasting

The exercising of water fasting, which involves going without foods and drinks that include energy and alternatively consuming just water, has an extended and sundry records this is reflective of the kind of human faith and way of life. Purification of frame and soul, illumination of spirit, and large health are all factors of the historical exercise that have deep roots.

This research takes us on an experience through the annals of water fasting, illuminating the cultural affects and modifications that have took place at a few level inside the centuries and conventional techniques of Life and concept.

Fasting as a Medical Practice in Ancient Greece

Ancient Greece, the birthplace of Western civilization, was no stranger to the exercising of fasting. Famous Greek scientific physician Hippocrates, from time to time called the "father of medicine," believed that fasting had medicinal houses.

His notion restoration can also moreover rise up extra speedy if the body needs to lighten up from the chronic pressure of digestion. Also stated within the Hippocratic Oath, a cornerstone textual content in medical ethics, are nutritional measures and the function of fasting in fitness maintenance.

Fasting as a Religious Practice in Ancient Mesopotamia and Egypt

Fasting changed into a crucial part of religious lifestyles for historic Mesopotamian and Egyptian cultures, going beyond its actual use in medical philosophy. Many humans believed that fasting helped cleanse every the frame and the soul. Fasting end up documented in historical sources as each an man or woman and network interest. Whole groups would possibly check instances of abstinence as a part of non secular ceremonies and rituals. Eastern Traditions and Spiritual Practices.

A Buddhist Perspective on Fasting and Its Role in Awakening.

As a non secular area, fasting has prolonged been important to Eastern faiths, specially Buddhism. In his pursuit of enlightenment, the legendary Buddhist founder Siddhartha Gautama famously fasted for an extended period of time. Buddhist monastic groups hold to workout conscious ingesting and intermittent fasting, despite the reality that he in the end gave up rigorous fasting for the Middle Way.

Fasting for Purity Rituals in Hinduism.

As a conventional non secular exercise, fasting is an vital a part of Hinduism's many ceremonies and fairs. Observance of fasting, or 'Vrat' or 'Upavasa,' isn't unusual inside the path of many fairs and particular sports. People count on it can cleanse the frame and soul, inspire energy of will, and result in benevolent spiritual forces. Partiality in fasting and nutritional regulations are commonplace practices in Hindu non secular traditions.

Taoism: Achieving Balance many of the Physical and the Ethereal

One way to supply concord to as a minimum one's body and soul is thru fasting, in step with Taoist philosophy. Moderation and fasting at normal intervals are harassed within the Tao Te Ching, a number one textual content of Taoism concept to were written by using the use of Laozi. According to this view, fasting allows purge pollution, repair electricity equilibrium, and bring one into harmony with the Tao's herbal order.Time of the Middle Ages and the Renaissance.

Christian Fasting in the center Ages

In mediaeval Christian faiths, fasting have end up furthermore significantly valued. It have become not unusual exercising to speedy for the duration of the holy seasons, along side Lent. As a form of non secular subject, fasting have become an crucial aspect of the lives of many organizations, which encompass monastic ones. Some humans concept that fasting from specific meals for set periods of time might motive them to extra humble and dedicated to their spirituality

Renaissance: A Time of Natural Healing and Fasting

During the Renaissance, while human beings were re-uncovered to the mind of the historical Greeks and Romans, the recovery houses of fasting have been another time brought to mild. Ancient clinical thinkers like Hippocrates inspired present day medical doctors to analyze fasting as a functionality natural treatment. Natural medicine, which emerged sooner or later of the Renaissance, started out out to examine fasting as part of its holistic technique to health.

Scientific Discovery and Contemporary Renewal.

Fasting as a Therapeutic Practice in the Nineteenth Century. The idea of fasting as a health benefit have come to be popular inside the 1800s. Proponents of fasting as a manner of bodily cleansing and contamination prevention included Presbyterian pastor and dietary reformer Sylvester Graham. There have become a surge in popularity for healthy consuming and extraordinary way of existence changes approximately this time, and Graham became a first-rate element in that.

Therapeutic Fasting Clinics within the Early twentieth Century

Due in huge element to the studies completed with the aid of Drs. John H. Tilden and Herbert M. Shelton, therapeutic fasting clinics started out out to spring up inside the early 1900s. These medical doctors encouraged fasting as a treatment alternative for various scientific issues. Fasting clinics sprang up, presenting supervised fasting regimens to folks who preferred to locate natural techniques to cope with chronic illnesses. Research on Fasting and Scientific Exploration within the Mid to Late 20th Century.

In the center to past due twentieth century, there has been a surge in scientific hobby in studying the physiological impacts of fasting. A fashion of studies have tested the effects of intermittent fasting on fitness and metabolism, together with one via Dr. Ancel Keys. A extra complicated information of fasting have emerge as viable while scientists started to deduce the molecular and cell techniques that underlie its benefits.

Views from the Present and the Spread of intermittent fasting's meteoric upward thrust. Intermittent fasting has been greater not unusual within the remaining numerous many years. The developing quantity of research demonstrating the health blessings of intermittent fasting has brought on its massive adoption with the aid of the usage of oldsters which may be looking to manipulate their weight and enhance their metabolic fitness. Some examples of these codecs of intermittent fasting embody the sixteen:8 method and the five:2 healthy eating plan.2.

The Wellness Movement and Popular Culture's Perception of Fasting.

Some fitness and health trends, such intermittent fasting and water fasting, have made manner into mainstream society. Fasting has entered the general public's attention due to severa influential assets, consisting of books, documentaries, and movie star endorsements of the exercising for fitness reasons. People seeking out a extra structured approach to fasting have additionally pushed growth inside the huge fashion of fasting retreats and wellness centers that offer supervised fasting instructions.

Final Thoughts: An Age-Old Custom in a Contemporary Setting.

Water fasting has a rich data that spans many disciplines and eras, which includes conventional medication, religious practices, and clinical inquiry. Throughout human facts, fasting has been an important part of many religious and philosophical practices, from the spiritual observances of the East to the philosophical writings of the historical Greek physicians. This historical exercise of water fasting is a timeless tool for holistic health that transcends cultural obstacles and echoes down the corridors of human statistics. As we negotiate the problems of modern-day lifestyles, it's miles critical to understand it in a contemporary context, manner to the ancient element of view.

Fasting in Islam

In Islam, fasting is known as "Sawm," and it has an extended past this is going lower lower back to religious traditions. The custom comes from the Quran, this is Islam's holy ebook. It says that the month of Ramadan is a holy time to fast. Fasting has an extended facts in Islam. It commenced in the seventh century, whilst Allah spoke to the Prophet Muhammad and informed him to fast all through the lunar month of Ramadan.

Muslims everywhere in the international fast from sunrise till nightfall, due to this they do not devour, drink, smoke, or do some thing else that is wrong. The speedy allows human beings come to be more spiritually natural, more self-disciplined, and in addition compassionate in the direction of oldsters that are in need. The month is remembered because the most effective on the identical time because the number one terms of the Quran have been validated to Prophet Muhammad.

In Islam, fasting is more than truely now not consuming or eating. It moreover way doing greater prayer, notion, and acts of kindness.

This culture from the past brings Muslims spherical the sector together and is a time of deep willpower, self-mirrored image, and community help. The past of fasting in Islam shows that this holy exercising has a deep spiritual this means that in an effort to in no way fade.

Understanding the similarities and versions amongst Water Fasting, Intermittent Fasting and Dry Fasting.

Intermittent Fasting

In the workout of intermittent fasting, one alternates amongst times of ingesting and durations of fasting, with the fasting durations frequently lasting among sixteen and 24 hours. For the duration of the fasting segment, this technique does allow the intake of beverages which includes water, tea, and brilliant drinks that don't include power.

Water Fasting

On the opportunity hand, water fasting is a exercising that involves consuming not some thing however water for a predetermined quantity of time, which can regularly range anywhere from twenty-four hours to numerous days. The exercise of water fasting need to be achieved with caution and underneath the steerage of a healthcare expert because it has the capacity to have massive affects on the body. It is important to emphasize that this is the case.

Dry Fasting

The maximum stringent shape of fasting is referred to as dry fasting, and it consists of restricting both meals and water intake for a predetermined quantity of time this is stated. When it involves the bulk of people, this technique is not advocated because of the truth it can result in awesome health issues and dehydration.

Focusing in your eating and fasting home windows is a notable deal much much less complex whilst you exercising intermittent fasting. You will exercise fasting for a predetermined time body, the length of that would range. For the period of this era, you are not allowed to consume any food or liquids other than water. In this form of water speedy, you could satisfactory eat water at some point of the fast. However, excellent methods for intermittent fasting will will let you drink black coffee and tea, provided which you do no longer upload any sweeteners, regardless of whether or now not or not or not they'll be low in power. Individuals should engage in water fasting on their personal, and it is a shape of detox diet regime that need to be approached with warning. The following are the similarities and versions among water fasting and intermittent fasting:

An powerful method for reaching weight loss further to preferred fitness and nicely-being is the workout of intermittent fasting. It can help in the law of blood sugar, boost up the metabolism, and decrease levels of cholesterol.

When it entails detox diets, water fasting is a shape of weight-reduction plan that should be addressed with caution due to the reality it could be risky over the path in their length. Although it has the capacity to stimulate autophagy and resource in illness prevention, it should now not be completed for an extended time body without the assistance of a scientific professional.

During water fasting, you are first rate allowed to devour water. On the alternative hand, in the direction of intermittent fasting, you're allowed to have non-caloric drinks which incorporates espresso or tea for the duration of your fasting intervals. This is the number one difference among water fasting and intermittent fasting.

Fasting on water ought to make the chance of getting orthostatic hypotension better, and it is able to moreover make sure illnesses that are already gift, on the facet of gout, even more immoderate. Be wonderful to are attempting to find the advice of a licensed medical practitioner in advance than beginning a water fast.

The preference amongst water fasting and intermittent fasting is one that need to be made based totally definitely mostly on your ambitions and the modern-day nation of your fitness. While water fasting can be considered as part of an intermittent fasting technique or under the advice of a scientific professional, intermittent fasting may be a extra sustainable desire for long-time period health and nicely-being advantages from a health and fitness attitude.

Chapter 2: The Health Benefits Of Water Fasting

One of the maximum enormous advantages of water fasting is that it is able to help in inducing a nation of nutritional ketosis. This is the usa in which your body stops the usage of glucose (carbohydrates and exceptional candies) as a delivery of electricity and alternatively uses fat as a delivery of power.

Fasting on water can also have a number of fitness advantages, in conjunction with the subsequent:

It aids short weight loss

Fasting with water permits people shed pounds extra brief thru a number of really one in all a type processes. While someone is fasting, their body is going right into a country known as ketosis, in which they transition from the usage of glucose as a deliver of electricity to breaking down fats that they have saved. The acceleration of fats burning that consequences from this metabolic shift contributes to the quick lack of weight. An more gain of water fasting is that it consequences in a calorie deficit for the purpose that absence of food consumption forces the frame to attract upon its very very own internal electricity reserves.

A further benefit of water fasting is that it impacts hormonal stability, reducing insulin degrees and growing insulin sensitivity. Reduced insulin ranges inspire the breakdown of fats garage, while extended insulin sensitivity contributes to more effective usage of strength whilst it is present. Additionally, the technique modulates starvation hormones like ghrelin and leptin, which enables to suppress desire and strengthens the capacity to paste to a regimen that restricts the form of power consumed.

A further detail that contributes to fast weight loss sooner or later of water fasting is the discount of water retention, the detoxing that takes vicinity through autophagy, and the highbrow modifications that stand up in ingesting conduct. On the possibility hand, it's far vital to approach water fasting with caution, making sure which you are correctly hydrated and searching for the help of a expert so that you can reduce the capacity risks which can be associated with extended durations of calorie limit.

It enables in improving cardiovascular health features

There are huge advantages for cardiovascular health from water fasting. It adjustments one-of-a-kind components of the cardiovascular device and improves modern-day fitness.

Blood strain happening, which may be very vital for coronary heart health, has been linked to the exercising. Cutting decrease again on calories even as fasting and making insulin art work higher together to decorate blood vessel characteristic, which lowers each systolic and diastolic blood pressure. This decrease is specifically useful for human beings with excessive blood stress as it lowers the risk of coronary heart problems.

Fasting moreover has an exceptional effect on lipid degrees, which results in a more healthy lipid profile. Total cholesterol, LDL

ldl cholesterol (additionally known as "terrible" ldl ldl cholesterol), and triglycerides can all flow down at the equal time as you fast on water, constant with studies. At the equal time, HDL ldl ldl cholesterol (the "real" ldl ldl ldl cholesterol) can also rise, which lowers the danger of atherosclerosis and coronary coronary heart ailment.

One more gain of water fasting is that it makes insulin paintings better, that is closely related to coronary coronary heart fitness. When insulin resistance is dwindled, the body is better able to manage blood sugar levels. This lowers the hazard of metabolic syndrome and the hazard of coronary coronary coronary heart illness, stroke, and type 2 diabetes.

Chronic infection, that may be a incredible cause of heart disease, additionally can be handled thru water fasting. Fasting starts offevolved offevolved offevolved a procedure referred to as autophagy, which permits do away with damaged cells and lowers infection within the frame as a whole. This makes the surroundings better for coronary heart fitness. The functionality to manipulate your weight, it is an important a part of coronary heart health, is advanced via water fasting. Creating a caloric stability and frightening the frame to apply fats as gasoline assist people shed pounds, it really is proper for his or her coronary heart health and lowers ldl ldl cholesterol and blood pressure.

Fasting has additionally been associated with higher endothelium characteristic, it really is essential for keeping blood vessels healthful. Improved endothelial function allows blood vessels nicely open and close, which lets in appropriate blood float and lowers the chance of artery stiffness and coronary heart issues.

It permits growth highbrow clarity

One important detail of the highbrow and physiological influences of water fasting is its have an effect on on mind clarity. There are a number of techniques that beautify attention all through a water speedy, wherein human beings drink first-class water and do not devour or drink anything with electricity.

The induction of ketosis is one of the important reasons why water fasting improves highbrow clarity. In the absence of food, the body enters a metabolic u . S . Whilst it begins to use its saved fats for gasoline, resulting within the production of ketone our bodies. When those ketones bypass the blood-thoughts barrier, they provide the mind with an trade strength supply that it can depend on. Some research have proven that ketones can boom cognitive function, which in turn improves highbrow clarity, and may simply have neuroprotective effects.

The mind's neurotransmitter stability may be tormented by fasting. Fasting causes a rise inside the neurotransmitter dopamine, that's involved in motivation and popularity; this, in flip, contributes to heightened consciousness and highbrow clarity. The protein brain-derived neurotrophic detail (BDNF) allows in neuronal improvement and protection, and fasting may additionally moreover have an impact on its ranges. Memory, mastering, and cognitive characteristic are all stronger even as BDNF levels are true sufficient.

Negative effects on cognitive feature and deterioration in memory had been associated with continual infection. By stimulating autophagy, the body's method of getting rid of damaged cells and converting them with new, healthful ones, water fasting enables lessen contamination. An environment that promotes top thoughts normal performance and mental clarity is one surrender end result of this irritation lower. The fourth element is an advanced mind-derived neurotrophic detail, or BDNF.

One of the maximum essential elements in keeping thoughts fitness and cognitive characteristic is BDNF, and studies has showed that fasting can enhance its manufacturing. BDNF is concerned in synaptic plasticity, the mind's ability to exchange and create new connections, and it furthermore permits in neuronal increase and protection. Mood, cognitive common basic performance, and fashionable intellectual clarity are all honestly correlated with progressed BDNF levels.

Cells are able to soak up glucose from the bloodstream extra successfully after a water fast, which will boom insulin sensitivity. The thoughts makes use of glucose for energy, as a end result that is vital for brain function. Fasting improves insulin sensitivity, which in flip maintains a normal and managed glucose supply to the thoughts, protective it from fluctuations that might reason highbrow haze and impaired hobby.

Clearer wondering is a factor effect of water fasting that has psychological roots as properly. Practicing energy of thoughts and area all through fasting could probably help one become extra privy to their environment and sharpen their hobby. People who rapid from water typically find out that they end up more self-aware, which in flip permits them higher recognize their non-public concept methods and preserve intellectual readability.

Finally, there are a number of procedures in which water fasting improves brain clarity. The physiological adjustments introduced approximately via water fasting provide a extraordinary putting for maximum dependable cognitive feature. These adjustments embody the thoughts's progressed production of BDNF, neurotransmitter modulation, contamination good buy, stepped forward insulin sensitivity, and ketosis, an opportunity gas supply for the thoughts. Fasting also allows with mental readability as it promotes intellectual area and mindfulness. Water fasting, like every fitness workout, calls for warning; humans with gift scientific troubles should workout greater caution, live properly hydrated, and spot a healthcare professional in advance than beginning the short.

Helps in reductions of cravings

Some human beings locate that water fasting lets in them control their urges, specially for awful materials. This is how water fasting changes cravings:

Water fasting allows maintain starvation chemical substances like ghrelin and leptin in take a look at. Ghrelin, that is now and again called the "starvation hormone," makes you hungry. Water fasting has been demonstrated to lower its quantities. At the identical time, fasting may additionally growth quantities of leptin, the hormone that tells the body it's far full. Because of this natural stability, humans do not need to devour as masses, because of this they do now not have as many cravings.

Insulin sensitivity is raised through water fasting, which makes it tons less hard for cells to take glucose from the bloodstream. This increase in insulin sensitivity permits keep blood sugar ranges constant, keeping off the quick rises and falls that may make you need sugary or high-carbohydrate additives. Water fasting reduces the physiological triggers which could motive cravings via the use of giving cells a extra ordinary and controlled supply of strength.

It takes willpower and place to do a water fast. Deliberately no longer eating for a positive amount of time builds intellectual manage that can be used to make meals alternatives after the fasting period is over. People frequently say that they may be greater aware about their dating with meals, which lets in them inform the difference amongst actual hunger and emotional or ordinary urges.

It's feasible that water fasting can assist reset your taste buds. People's taste buds may additionally moreover moreover end up greater touchy all through fasting because of the truth they do now not consume sure matters. Because of this sensitivity, you might not need as many overly candy or pretty processed foods. This have to make it easier to start ingesting greater healthy and combat cravings for much less wholesome food.

Helps in kidney cleaning and feature

Water lets in the tool of diuresis, which is an vital part of kidney characteristic and is managed by means of way of a complicated set of physiological systems. In terms of medicine, this is the way it works:

The first step takes place within the kidney corpuscle, in a small organization of capillaries commonplace like a ball. This business enterprise is known as the glomerulus. The afferent arteriole brings blood into the glomerulus. Blood consists of water. Lots of water and dissolved materials, like glucose, salts, and waste, are driven into the Bowman's pill through the immoderate pressure in the glomerulus.

The filtrate, it's a liquid mix of water and one-of-a-kind solutes, goes into the renal tubules and starts offevolved the device of making urine. Some topics, like glucose, amino acids, and salts, are taken lower back into the bloodstream via the proximal convoluted tubule.

Limbs of the Loop of Henle that go down and up. The filtrate then is going into the Henle loop, in which it is focused and diluted even greater. The lowering limb lets water go with the go with the flow out, which makes the filtrate greater targeted. The ascending limb moves ions round, which lets in the attention gradient inside the medulla.

The filtrate that has been focused goes into the accumulating tubes. Antidiuretic hormone (ADH), a hormone, can be very essential in this case. If the frame desires to maintain water, ADH makes the walls of the collecting tubes extra porous just so water can skip thru them and again into the bloodstream. When the frame wants to eliminate more water, ADH degrees drop. This makes the accumulating tubes lots much less permeable to water.

The final step is the removal of urine. Depending at the body's desires, the urine moves via the renal pelvis and down the ureter. It then shops inside the bladder until it's far emptied thru the urethra.

During the whole way, water may be very critical. Making extremely good you drink sufficient water makes sure that the glomerulus has enough fluid for filtering. This we should the kidneys get rid of waste and maintain the electrolyte stability. If you do not drink sufficient water, your pee will become more focused, that could make you much more likely to get kidney stones or wonderful problems together collectively along with your kidneys.

Enhance liver function and cleaning

There is proof that water fasting can help the frame put off pollutants through the use of helping its herbal structures, specifically the liver. In many techniques, water fasting could make the liver art work better. The liver is an vital a part of the frame's cleaning device.

When you nice drink water, your body goes proper into a kingdom referred to as ketosis, in which it uses fat stores for power. With this variation in metabolism, fats stores are used up, and pollution that have been saved in fatty tissue are released. When the ones poisons get into the body, the liver will be very important because it breaks them down and receives rid of them.

When you rapid, your liver goes via adjustments which could make it better at casting off pollution. The liver breaks down and neutralizes pollution, turning them into water-soluble chemical substances that the frame can remove thru pee or bile.

Oxidative pressure, that's associated with the body making dangerous free radicals, has been related to a decrease hazard of fasting. Toxins can building up because of oxidative stress. Fasting in a roundabout way lets in cleaning by means of the usage of decreasing this pressure.

When you fast, you provide your digestive machine a harm. This we could it relaxation and use its electricity to clean out your frame. By lowering the quantity of pollution that come in from meals, this spoil can help the liver and exclusive structures that easy the body paintings better.

Getting rid of saved waste: When the frame goes proper proper right into a fasting country, it starts offevolved to attention on doing away with waste. This includes removing poisons and metabolic waste that may have built up in unique organs and tissues.

It Increase power degree

There is proof that water fasting can provide you with plenty greater electricity. It is a completely particular way to refresh your body and mind. The body is going right into a country referred to as ketosis whilst it does no longer consume for a while. During this time, it receives most of its power from stored fat. This alternate in metabolism makes the body's strength use extra green, giving it a fuel deliver that lasts longer and stays normal.

Water fasting moreover lets in the frame make ketone our our bodies, which might be used as an opportunity food deliver, specially for the thoughts. People recognize that ketones can offer a dependable and effective supply of electricity and improve interest and clarity of perception. In addition, stopping digestion for a quick time we have to the body use energy that might commonly be used to interrupt down food for repair and renewal. During fasting, cellular autophagy is speeded up, which lets in take away damaged cells and cellular additives, which improves the overall health of cells.

In giant, most humans say that they have masses extra power in the course of and after a water rapid. However, anyone's revel in may be a little distinct. This is because of the adjustments in metabolism and cell regeneration that occur because of this vintage exercise.

It lets in in strengthening of the immune tool

Water fasting can beautify the immune machine by way of manner of the usage of some of routes that artwork together. Autophagy is an vital element to bear in mind due to the reality it is a mobile technique that begins offevolved while you fast. The approach of autophagy receives rid of damaged or defective cells and factors of cells. This makes the immune device more potent and faster.

Inflammation is a natural system that lets in the immune tool fight off infections and harm. Water fasting also can make contamination pass down. Fasting lowers prolonged contamination, which makes the body a higher place for immune cells to artwork at their high-quality.

There is likewise evidence that water fasting may be proper for the micro organism within the intestine. A balanced and sundry bacteria is critical for immune health as it allows the immune device observe the difference amongst chemical materials which can be risky and chemical materials that aren't.

The body prioritizes using power for essential obligations while you fast, directing resources toward immune system capabilities like making immune cells. This alternate in metabolism makes wonderful that the immune device gets the terrific resource at some stage in the fasting segment.

Slow down growing older and increase life expectancy

In many techniques, water fasting can slow down the developing older manner and make humans live longer. Autophagy is a technique that helps remove damaged elements of cells. Fasting will boom autophagy, which might also moreover assist cells renew themselves and sluggish down the developing older approach. Fasting additionally lowers reactive stress, because of this that it lowers the producing of dangerous unfastened radicals that might accelerate mobile harm and growing older.

Fasting improves the feature of mitochondria, which in flip makes power production greater inexperienced in cells. This is good for the fitness of cells as a whole. Additionally, regular exercising increases insulin sensitivity, which lowers the chance of getting insulin resistance and type 2 diabetes, every of which can be often associated with residing a longer life.

Sirtuins are proteins that can be activated via fasting. These proteins are connected to living longer. Sirtuins help manage how cells work, and turning them on would probable make people stay longer.

Chronic contamination is a big a part of growing older, so fasting's anti-inflammatory advantages are very essential. It's possible that fasting can decrease irritation, which can make age-associated illnesses a bargain less severe.

All this are functionality benefits of fasting inside the subsequent chapter we're able to communicate the protection measures, risks connected, beauty of folks that must now not embark on fasting and a way to put together for at the same time as setting out water fasting.

Chapter 3: Getting Prepared

Safety Measures suggestions to remember in advance than embarking on water fasting

When starting water fast, it is vital to offer cautious attention to the scenario and stick with protection strategies that allow you to hold one's fitness for the duration of the length of the quick. When starting a water fast, it's miles essential to take the subsequent precautions to make certain your protection:

Consultation with Professionals inside the Healthcare Sector

A consultation alongside facet your healthcare company needs to take area preceding to beginning any fasting everyday. This is extremely crucial, in particular if you have any pre-cutting-edge clinical conditions, are presently taking any capsules, or fall into any of the areas in which fasting ought to doubtlessly harm you.

An Individualized Strategy:

You should collaborate with a professional nutritionist or a healthcare practitioner if you need to enlarge a customized fasting technique that is tailored on your present day country of health, your man or woman goals, and your way of lifestyles.]

An Evaluation in advance than the Fasting.

Before beginning a fasting recurring, it's miles critical to go through a radical health assessment, which need to embody blood finding out, in case you want to decide your modern-day kingdom of health. This may be helpful in figuring out potential risks and guiding the technique that is taken to fasting.

Techniques for Hydration.

Plan a technique for staying hydrated. To avoid being dehydrated while fasting, it's miles critical to consume an good enough amount of water. While you're fasting, you need to make sure which you are eating water that has been filtered and is simple.

Electrolyte Balance.

Ensure that the electrolyte balance is monitored and maintained. To prevent imbalances which could result in problems, it's far critical to consider the opportunity of introducing electrolyte-wealthy liquids or dietary supplements, specifically during prolonged fasts.

Gradual Approach.

If that is your first time fasting, you want to remember beginning out slowly. Before trying longer water fasts, it is advocated to start with shorter fasting periods, including intermittent fasting which may be shorter in length.

Make an try and educate your self.

Gain an know-how of the functionality advantages and risks related to water fasting. Familiarize your self with the signs and symptoms and signs of issues and be aware about the right times to break the fast or seeking out clinical treatment.

Keeping an eye fixed constant regular on each someone's bodily and mental health.

While you're fasting, it's miles vital to maintain a close to eye on every your physical and emotional fitness. It is vital to take note of any signs and symptoms and signs that are not conventional, and in case you are experiencing top notch pain, you need to harm your fast and speak with a scientific practitioner.

Avoid Engaging in Strenuous Activities.

When you are fasting, you want to refrain from conducting strenuous physical sports. In order in your frame to modify to the fasting situation without overstressing itself, you have to offer it the rest it dreams.

Be conscious as you damage the quick.

Breaking the fast need to be achieved in a sluggish and careful way. If you need to avoid digestive issues, you need to begin with meals which can be easy to digest after which frequently upload more complicated food.

Social Assistance.

You need to let your family and friends apprehend approximately your plan to speedy. The presence of a guide gadget may be effective, particularly if the human beings in that device are aware of your dreams and are able to provide encouragement.

Plan for Emergencies.

In the event of an emergency, you should have a plan. Be aware of the places of the nearest scientific centers, and permit someone close to you apprehend approximately your desire to speedy in order that they may provide help within the occasion that it is required. It is crucial to maintain in mind that specific people have special reactions to fasting, and what works for one character might not be suitable for some special. It is critical to make safety a top priority and to are trying to find the assist of experts as a way to make sure a super enjoy on the equal time as fasting on the identical time as concurrently minimizing the dangers that may be worried.

People who can't speedy

There are many fitness advantages to water fasting for plenty humans. However, there are some groups of folks that ought to be cautious with fasting or stay faraway from it altogether. Some of these are:

People Who Already Have Certain Medical Conditions.

Before trying water fasting, individuals who have already got diabetes, coronary heart ailment, kidney troubles, or specific long-time period medical situations have to talk to their clinical doctors. Fasting might probably alternate the amount of medication you want and your health in famous.

Women who are pregnant or breastfeeding.

Women who are pregnant or nursing need extra vitamins to keep themselves and their babies healthy. Because fasting may want to make you lose vitamins, it isn't an splendid concept at some point of these times.

Teenagers and children.

Bodies which are regardless of the reality that growing have precise nutritional desires, and fasting can also additionally get inside the manner of right improvement and boom. Teenagers and children shouldn't do water fasting with out a scientific doctor's steering.

People who've had consuming troubles within the beyond.

People who've had anorexia nervosa or bulimia within the past have to not speedy due to the reality it could purpose them to eat extra poorly or make their modern-day situations worse.

People over the age of sixty five.

Some older human beings might also moreover moreover have particular dietary desires, and fasting without the proper help can leave them quick on vitamins. Before suggesting that older human beings rapid, their present day fitness and scientific statistics ought to be taken into consideration.

People who're underweight or malnourished.

People who're already underweight or terrible have to now not fast because of the truth it could cause them to lose even extra weight and now not get enough nutrients.

People with Low Blood Pressure.

People with low blood stress have to be cautious when they speedy because of the truth it may lower their blood pressure. If you do now not drink enough water even as fasting, this situation may additionally moreover worsen.

People who are vulnerable to hypoglycemia.

People who have had hypoglycemia (low blood sugar) inside the beyond also can have worse signs and symptoms and signs and symptoms and signs at the same time as fasting. This is at the same time as it is very crucial to preserve a watch on blood sugar tiers.

People who have highbrow fitness troubles.

People who have already got some intellectual fitness troubles, like disappointment, anxiety, or bipolar sickness, can be damage with the resource of the emotional and mental stress that includes fasting. Fasting can change your temper and strength tiers, that could make intellectual fitness issues worse.

People who're taking medications.

Some drugs might also furthermore want to be interested in food whenever. People who're taking drug treatments for prolonged-time period situations, psychiatric issues, or unique health troubles ought to speak to their clinical health practitioner before fasting because of the reality the timing of after they take their medicines may also want to be modified.

People who have troubles with their intestines.

If you have got a digestive hassle like inflammatory bowel disease, irritable bowel syndrome, or persistent gastritis, your symptoms may also additionally moreover get worse even as you rapid. Not having meals can also aggravate the digestive system, that can cause pain or distinct problems.

Players or People Who Are Very Active.

People who do excessive bodily sports activities sports or game enthusiasts who use pretty a few power may additionally additionally discover it hard to preserve up their everyday normal performance while water fasting. Getting enough meals is crucial for keeping up your electricity and assisting your body work at its first rate.

People who have been dehydrated or had electrolyte problems in the beyond.

Fasting, specifically if you don't drink enough water, could make you dehydrated and throw off your electrolytes. People who've had those kinds of problems within the past, like kidney problems or a bent for chemical imbalances, want to be careful and drink enough water.

People who've hassle drowsing or insomnia.

Changing the manner you eat, particularly even as you are fasting, should make it hard to sleep. People who have trouble dozing or sleeplessness want to be aware of how fasting would possibly have an effect at the excellent and length in their sleep.

People who are touchy or allergic.

The manner the frame reacts to allergens can also moreover additionally alternate whilst you speedy. People who understand they may be allergic to or touchy to sure materials want to don't forget how the ones elements might possibly have an effect on their immune device and stylish fitness.

People with Certain Mental Health Conditions.

The emotional and highbrow pressure that includes fasting may be worse for people with excessive first-class highbrow health conditions, like unhappiness, tension, or bipolar illness. Fasting can exchange your temper and energy levels, which can make intellectual fitness issues worse.

People who are taking capsules.

Some drug treatments may also moreover need to be considering meals whenever. People who're taking drug treatments for extended-term conditions, psychiatric problems, or unique fitness problems need to speak to their health practitioner before fasting because of the fact the timing of after they take their medicinal drugs can also moreover need to be changed.

People with Digestive Problems.

People with digestive troubles like inflammatory bowel sickness, irritable bowel syndrome, or continual gastritis may additionally additionally have worse signs once they speedy. Not having meals may moreover get worse the digestive device, which could cause pain or precise troubles. Players or

People who have been dehydrated or had electrolyte problems within the beyond.

Fasting, especially in case you do no longer drink enough water, could make you dehydrated and throw off your electrolytes. People who've had the ones kinds of issues inside the past, like kidney problems or a dishonest for chemical imbalances, have to be cautious and drink sufficient water.

Prior to taking off a water fasting interest, persons who fall into any of these corporations have to see healthcare practitioners to take a look at that fasting is properly best with their specific fitness conditions. It is crucial to continuously supply pinnacle priority to safety and nicely-being whilst thinking of any shape of fasting or substantial dietary changes.

Potential Danger of Fasting

Water fasting, if not undertaken with warning, may also gift possible dangers and health issues. Prior to taking off a water fasting undertaking, it's far essential to personal information of those possibly limitations:

Insufficient intake of important nutrients.

Prolonged bouts of water fasting can result in inadequate consumption of important nutrients. Insufficient consumption of critical vitamins and minerals can reason imbalances in the frame, which could have negative results on many physiological tactics.

Electrolyte imbalances.

Extended periods of fasting can result in disturbances in electrolyte ranges, that can intervene with the everyday operation of the coronary coronary heart, muscle tissues, and neurons. Sodium, potassium, and other electrolytes play a essential role in retaining mobile equilibrium.

Dehydration.

Insufficient consumption of water during fasting can result in dehydration. Dehydration can exert strain at the kidneys and prevent their general overall performance, potentially resulting in problems.

Orthostatic hypotension

Abstaining from meals can bring about a lower in blood strain, which could result in orthostatic hypotension. This syndrome can cause signs and symptoms together with vertigo, syncope, or accidental falls, specifically whilst assuming an upright characteristic.

Muscle Atrophy

Prolonged fasting can bring about the catabolism of muscle mass to provide strength. This can lead to muscular atrophy and a decline in everyday physical energy.

Cognitive impairment.

The cognitive characteristic can be laid low with dehydration and meals shortages that arise for the duration of fasting, resulting in stressful situations in focus, memory, and preference-making.

Refeeding Syndrome

Refeeding Syndrome refers to a probably lifestyles-threatening state of affairs which can arise while an individual who's malnourished or starved begins offevolved to devour another time.

It can arise if a brief is ended too rapid or if a huge amount of meals is fed on. This circumstance involves disturbances in electrolyte degrees and has the functionality to be deadly.

Gastrointestinal Problems.

Abstaining from food over a term might probably reason gastrointestinal problems along side nausea, constipation, or diarrhea. Sudden reintroduction of food can get worse those problems.

Impaired Immune System.

Prolonged fasting should probably probably impair the immune device, rendering the body extra liable to illnesses.

Hormonal Imbalances.

Fasting might also have an impact on hormonal equilibrium, which may additionally additionally bring about disturbances within the menstrual cycle for ladies or modifications in reproductive hormones.

Exacerbation of pre-modern conditions.

Individuals who have pre-present scientific troubles which includes diabetes, coronary coronary coronary heart disease, or kidney issues may additionally moreover enjoy a deterioration of their situations at the identical time as fasting.

Psychological Consequences.

Fasting can bring about mental symptoms which encompass mood fluctuations, impatience, anxiety, or an immoderate focus on consuming. Individuals who've previously professional eating troubles are prone to relapse.

Prudent deliberation is critical on the identical time as embarking on water fasting, specially for humans with preexisting health issues or precise risk elements. To mitigate those functionality issues, it's miles in reality beneficial to are attempting to find suggest from healthcare professionals, gradually introduce fasting, and often screen health signs. It is essential to usually deliver top priority to safety. If you are unsure, it's miles encouraged to attempting to find guidance from a expert healthcare professional before accomplishing any form of fasting.

Chapter 4: Common Mistakes Throughout Water Fasting

If you need to make sure a remarkable and a success experience at the same time as fasting on water, it's critical to technique the technique with careful attention. Here are a few not unusual mistakes human beings make whilst fasting on water, together with awesome reasons that will help you keep away from them:

Lack of Hydration.

Mistake: Fatigue, vertigo, and dehydration can quit result from no longer drinking enough water in the course of fasting.

Solution: The solution is to drink sufficient water each day and possibly even upload electrolyte-rich beverages or herbal teas to preserve yourself hydrated and balanced.

Medical Consultation Absence.

Mistake: Fasting with out first speakme to a health practitioner may be risky, particularly for human beings who have already were given health issues.

Solution: The solution is to make sure you visit a scientific physician very well in advance than fasting. Talk to your clinical clinical physician about your fasting method and medical records to make sure it suits your precise desires.

Fasting Schedules That Are Too Ambitious.

Mistake: If you've got had been given in no manner fasted for an extended time body before or have now not prepared for it, it can be difficult.

Solution: The solution is to ease into fasting through doing shorter cycles (intermittent fasting is one example) after which developing the time as your frame adjusts. Take it clean and be aware about your frame.

Inadequate Nutrient Consumption Prior to Fasting.

Mistake: Premature fasting because of a lack of nutrient-dense meals intake is a commonplace mistake.

Solution: The answer is to make certain you get sufficient of the nutrients and minerals you need with the beneficial resource of ingesting a balanced weight loss program inside the days previous up to the fast. For tailor-made recommendations, it could be useful to talk with a nutritionist.

Limited Preparation.

Mistake: Nutritional imbalances and odd ingesting styles may cease stop end result from fasting with out a proper plan.

Solution: A thorough fasting plan, which embody techniques for getting into and leaving the fast, need to be prepared. Make a time table in your meals, preserve tune of how your body reacts, and change it up as you pass.

Ignoring Nonverbal Cues.

Mistake: It's risky to ignore symptoms and symptoms and signs of exhaustion, lightheadedness, or excessive ache.

Solution: The solution is to pay near hobby to the manner you feel for the duration of fasting. Consider breaking the short and consulting a medical doctor if you stumble upon excessive ache or concerning symptoms and signs and symptoms and signs and symptoms.

Poor Management of Electrolytes

Mistake: Electrolyte imbalance, that can motive troubles like palpitations or muscle cramps, ought to not be overlooked.

Solution: To healing this, consume greater food which might be rich in electrolytes or take electrolyte dietary supplements, specially during prolonged fasts. Keep a close to eye on the whole thing and cope with any discrepancies right away.

Indulging Too Much When Cutting Off Food.

Mistake: Having a big or risky meal right after fasting need to lead to gastrointestinal troubles and pain.

Solution: The answer is to break the fast with modest meals which is probably rich in vitamins. Reestablishing regular ingesting styles can assist alleviate digestive ache. It's brilliant to start via specializing in ingredients which can be clean to digest.

Ditch the Idea of Emotional Health.

Mistake: Neglecting intellectual fitness whilst fasting can reason worry, mood swings, and a experience of deprivation, that is a mistake.

Solution: Make intellectual education a top precedence. Have an splendid outlook, be gift in the 2nd, and reap out to loved ones or experts for help even as you want it.

10. Disregarding Care after FAST.

Mistakes: Skipping the time after a short could affect how your frame adjusts, which could motive you to devour too much.

Solution: Reestablishing regular consuming styles need to be executed regularly. To gauge your frame's response, start with smaller quantities and consume more regularly. Be looking for signs and signs and signs of gastrointestinal distress and adjust your remedy plan consequently.

Individuals can maximize the safety and effectiveness in their water fasting experience thru addressing those not unusual issues and providing thorough answers. Prioritize your fitness, get expert advocate, and rapid with expertise and moderation.

Bursting Common Fasting Myths

Water fasting has garnered hobby due to its capacity health benefits, but there are various misconceptions surrounding this exercise. Here, we make clear a few commonplace misconceptions and shed light at the fact of water fasting:

Myth 1: Fasting Leads to Muscle Loss

Reality: In spite of the reality that extended fasting might also bring about a lack of a few muscle tissues, the body's primary supply of electricity for the duration of fasting is the fats that it has collected. After a fast, consuming an proper sufficient amount of protein and tasty in resistance education can help reduce the quantity of muscle that is misplaced.

Myth 2: Fasting causes a decrease in metabolic fee

Reality: The fact is that fasting for a short time frame can also first of all produce a discount in metabolic charge; though, this is a natural adaptive response. The findings of positive studies advise that intermittent fasting may not have a good sized effect on the overall metabolism, and it'd even turn out to be greater effective through the years.

Myth three: Fasting may also moreover result in deficiencies in some vitamins

Reality: Contrary to popular perception, fasting does not often bring about nutrient deficits when it's far accomplished with focus and via careful planning. It is possible to hold key nutrient ranges strong via ingesting enough quantities of food each earlier than and after fasting, further to with the aid of drinking enough water.

Myth 4: Fasting consequences in a weakened immune device

Reality: Despite the truth that prolonged fasting might also additionally additionally in short impair the immune device, intermittent fasting has the capability to have effects which can be beneficial to the immune machine. Periods of fasting that are each brief-term and everyday have the functionality to beautify immune characteristic via facilitating the removal of damaged cells.

Myth five: Fasting Causes Starvation Mode to Develop

Reality: The body does no longer input a "starvation mode" till it has lengthy beyond for a prolonged time period without ingesting any meals. Abstinence from water for a quick time frame does not elicit this reaction. Fasting reasons the body to transition to the usage of fats shops as a source of power, which contributes to the fee at which weight reduction takes location.

Myth 6: Everyone Can Benefit Equally from Fasting

Reality: The truth is that the outcomes of fasting variety from character to man or woman. One's reaction to fasting is stimulated thru a choice of things, which encompass their age, current-day health recognition, and way of lifestyles selections. It is crucial to are trying to find recommendation from a healthcare practitioner to make certain that fasting is suitable for the person's requirements.

Myth 7: Fasting detoxify the Body

Reality: There are herbal cleaning techniques that arise within the frame, and the liver and kidneys are basically liable for wearing them out. The idea of fasting as a cleansing useful resource is oversimplified, regardless of the fact that fasting can be beneficial to those methods. Hydration and preserving a healthy food regimen are of the most crucial factors of detoxing.

Myth 8: Fasting motives binge eating in a while

Reality: A conscious making plans approach and a slow transition returned to everyday meals can assist prevent binge consuming, despite the fact that some human beings may additionally furthermore revel in an boom of their appetite after a short. Fasting does no longer always encourage horrible consuming behavior; the choices and actions that an individual chooses to interact in are critical.

Myth nine: all and sundry can take part in fasting.

Reality: It is possible that those who are pregnant or breastfeeding, kids, humans who have particular fitness issues, or the ones who've a statistics of consuming troubles must now not have interaction in fasting. When identifying whether or not or no longer or now not some thing is suitable, it's far critical to visit a healthcare practitioner.

Myth 10: fasting will ensure weight loss.

Reality: The reality is that no matter the truth that fasting can help people shed kilos, the effects could likely variety considerably. Changes in weight are induced via a range of factors, such as an individual's metabolism, meals, and way of lifestyles in huge. Managing one's weight in a sustainable way requires taking a complete approach that is going beyond fasting.

Chapter 5: Harnessing The Power For Weight Loss

How to Use the Power of Water Fasting to Help You Lose Weight

People who need to lose weight in a healthy manner that lasts have discovered water fasting to be an appealing alternative. Not most effective is it remarkable for you bodily, however it additionally starts offevolved crucial biochemical techniques. According to this method, you ought to not eat or drink a few component with strength and ought to handiest drink water for a difficult and rapid amount of time, which can be everywhere from 24 hours to severa days or maybe weeks. Further studies is wanted to sincerely understand how water fasting allows people shed pounds. This can outstanding be finished via looking extra intently at the physiological adjustments that display up at some point of this time of beneficial calorie restrict.

1. The utilization of fats and the deficit of power.

Creating a calorie deficit is the unmarried maximum essential element that contributes to the weight loss consequences of water fasting. Internal reserves are utilized by the frame within the event that it does no longer acquire any outside assets of strength via the consumption of food. Within the begin tiers, glycogen stores are tired, which leads to a reduction in water weight. Nevertheless, due to the fact the fasting length keeps, the frame enters a situation of ketosis in the direction of this time. When the frame is on this metabolic u . S ., it begins offevolved breaking down fats that has been stored into ketone our our bodies, that are useful as an trade supply of energy. One of the maximum vital members to the massive weight reduction that may be located sooner or later of water fasting is the shift in the course of fat utilization.

2. An Increased Rate of Metabolic Activity.

A huge sort of research have cautioned that water fasting for a quick time body can also additionally additionally certainly boom metabolic rate, it's opposite to the not unusual belief that fasting slows down the metabolism. When there can be a loss of food, the frame reacts via developing the ranges of the hormone norepinephrine. Norepinephrine is a hormone that plays a thing within the activation of thermogenesis, this is the method with the beneficial aid of which the frame generates warmth and burns calories. By contributing to the acceleration of fats breakdown, this improved metabolic interest enables in the way of weight loss.

three. Decreased Insulin Levels and an Increased Sensitivity to Insulin.

There is evidence that fasting with water can lower insulin levels, it's an important hormone that performs a feature in controlling blood sugar levels and fats accumulation. In order to prevent the accumulation of greater fats, decrease insulin levels urge the frame to draw energy from its fats stores, which might be saved within the frame. Additionally, fasting improves insulin sensitivity, which in turn improves the body's ability to make effective use of insulin. This impact is particularly useful for humans who've insulin resistance or type 2 diabetes because of the truth it can reason higher manage of blood sugar tiers and higher management of weight.

4. Control of Appetite and the Maintenance of Hormonal Balance.

Water fasting has an effect at the hormonal signs which is probably associated with feelings of starvation and fullness. The hormone ghrelin, this is liable for boosting urge for meals, has an inclination to drop inside the course of intervals of fasting, which allows to make it less difficult to control hunger. On the opportunity component, there may be a possibility that leptin, the hormone that indicates fullness, must growth, as a way to further make contributions to the suppression of urge for meals. Individuals are capable of preserve a calorie deficit without experiencing extreme hunger due to this hormonal interaction, which makes it less complicated for them to stick to the fasting time desk.

five. Detoxification and the discount of water retention.

When the frame is fasting on water, it is going thru a manner referred to as autophagy, wherein it eliminates cells which is probably damaged or defective by using way of using breaking them down and disposing of them. This cleansing of the cells not most effective enables to hold regular fitness, but it moreover has the capacity to make contributions to a discount in infection. A quick drop in frame weight that extends past the dearth of fat or muscular tissues may be carried out by means of way of the workout of water fasting. This is due to the fact water fasting may moreover reason a lower in water retention.

6. Changes in Behaviours and Psychological Makeup.

Over and above the physiological components, water fasting has the capability to result in highbrow and behavioral adjustments which might be useful to weight loss. Mindfulness regarding ingesting patterns can be recommended via the deliberate act of abstaining from food from time to time. People regularly amplify a extra healthy dating with food because of becoming extra privy to the signs and symptoms and signs and signs and symptoms that propose at the same time as they may be hungry and at the same time as they'll be complete. Furthermore, the willpower and vicinity which can be superior at some point of water fasting can be carried over into positioned up-fast intervals, which could have an effect on an individual's prolonged-term ingesting choices.

Chapter 6: Autophagy And Cell Regeneration

The method of encouraging mobile regeneration via autophagy is a crucial problem in the context of water fasting, as it performs a large role in selling hooked up health and defensive in opposition to a whole lot of issues. Fasting on water is set up to this technique within the following manner:

The unique which means of the word "autophagy" comes from the Greek phrases "car," because of this "self," and "phagy," which means that that "ingesting." The device of autophagy can be understood as a self-cleansing mechanism that cells use to get rid of additives which may be broken or faulty. This approach facilitates to make certain that the health and integrity of the mobile is preserved.

The starting of autophagy is a crucial reaction that takes place at the same time as there are not any outside property of nutrients gift, which takes place even as one is fasting on water. Signaling pathways inside cells end up active due to the fact the frame transitions into a fasting u.S.A.. This activation sets off a series of activities that ultimately outcomes within the increase of autophagy. The mechanistic goal of rapamycin, frequently known as mTOR, is a protein kinase that plays a important function in regulating the development and metabolism of cells. It is one of the most vital gamers in this way. This lower in mTOR interest serves as a catalyst for the begin of autophagy, which occurs while a person is fasting.

The device of autophagy includes the development of specialized structures known as autophagosomes. These autophagosomes are answerable for engulfing and encasing cell components which can be destined to be degraded. After that, these autophagosomes combine with lysosomes, which may be cell organelles which might be whole of enzymes, which ultimately results inside the breakdown of the cloth that turn out to be ingested. The breakdown products which are produced as a cease result, at the side of amino acids and fatty acids, are able to being recycled and utilized by the cellular in order to generate strength and gather crucial mechanisms in the mobile.

The consequences of autophagy are not limited to the upkeep of cell systems; it additionally plays a big element within the adaptive responses to stress, it helps keep power homeostasis, and it adds to the body's defense in opposition to infections. In addition, the procedure of autophagy, which entails the removal of broken cell components, has been associated with a whole lot of fitness blessings. These advantages embody an extended lifespan in addition to a reduced hazard of growing excessive quality illnesses.

In essence, water fasting acts as a purpose for the sensitive dance of mobile self-purification that is taking vicinity. The gadget of autophagy, it definitely is a organic phenomena that now not best allows to cleanse and renew cells but additionally contributes to the general resilience and energy of the organism, is activated at the same time as the body accepts the brief absence of outside food.

In order to shed mild at the sensitive interaction amongst nutritional states and cellular upkeep, it's miles crucial to have an knowledge of the start of autophagy inside the route of fasting. This understanding well-known the terrific capability of the body to provoke self-renewal and version.

How Damaged Cells are handled within the route of Fasting

The manner of autophagy can be very critical for cell fitness as it helps cells eliminate damaged or malfunctioning elements. This complicated device works like a "clean-up group" inner cells, ensuring that the surroundings stays honestly proper for them to art work well.

Different components and proteins inside the mobile do unique jobs each day. Some of those factors of cells might also get damaged or save you operating proper through the years because of things like oxidative stress, the environment, or ordinary put on and tear. This is wherein autophagy is to be had in.

Autophagy is the technique via which cells make unique systems referred to as autophagosomes. These systems wrap spherical and enclose the damaged or non-running additives of cells which can be going to be removed. Once they will be enclosed, the ones autophagosomes be part of with lysosomes, which may be factors of cells that encompass enzymes that could wreck down the subjects inner them.

In this manner, the destroyed factors are broken down into their simple building blocks, like fatty acids and amino acids. These damaged-down materials can then be reused via the cellular to make strength or to construct new, wholesome mobile structures.

Autophagy is an important device for maintaining cells wholesome as it receives rid of damaged elements. It stops the accumulation of possibly dangerous mobile particles, which, if now not stopped, need to stop cells from running properly and motive some of fitness issues. Basically, autophagy is a simply essential first-rate manipulate machine inner cells that helps them final longer and keep running at their exceptional.

Disease Prevention thru Autophagy During Water Fasting

Because it may enhance autophagy, water fasting is becoming more and more famous as a manner to keep away from sickness via supporting cells easy themselves and grow to be stronger. Autophagy is a manner that starts offevolved offevolved in cells whilst you fast. It is a key a part of shielding the frame toward many illnesses.

One important vicinity of effect is preventing most cancers. The technique of autophagy keeps an eye fixed fixed on matters and gets rid of any broken or changed cells that would change into maximum cancers. By getting rid of these unusual cells, autophagy lowers the threat of cells growing out of manage and turning cancerous, which permits guard within the route of maximum cancers.

Autophagy has an effect on many ailments, especially neurodegenerative illnesses, further to stopping most cancers. In diseases like Alzheimer's and Parkinson's, autophagy allows get rid of superb proteins that constructing up in neurons. This improves the fitness of cells and might gradual the improvement or spread of those illnesses.

It's moreover crucial to recollect that autophagy enables combat infections. Autophagy allows the body fight off infections with the useful resource of making it much less hard to get rid of pathogens, viruses, and excellent risky microorganisms. During a water rapid, this innate immune response is mainly crucial because better tiers of autophagy help take away intracellular invaders brief.

Metabolic diseases, like diabetes, may additionally benefit from the strategies that autophagy stops illnesses. Getting rid of elements of cells that do not art work right, in particular in tissues that help control metabolism, makes cells artwork higher and can help avoid or deal with metabolic troubles.

Basically, water fasting triggers autophagy, it's a protection tool that allows put off broken cells, atypical proteins, and special topics that would be risky to mobile health. Because of those many outcomes, water fasting may be visible as an entire way to keep away from getting ill. It can help us apprehend how vitamins, cellular care, and the frame's natural capacity to fight off diseases all paintings together.

Keeping and improving mobile characteristic

With its functionality to start autophagy, water fasting is a key part of keeping and improving cellular characteristic, making sure that cells work at their great although they have no outdoor nutrients. This complicated approach of cells renewing and cleaning themselves enables the frame cope with strain, making cells more potent and improving fitness in present day.

When you most effective drink water at some point of a water fast, your frame has to use its non-public strength stores as a substitute of having nutrients from meals or beverages. When you fast, your frame begins a technique known as autophagy. This enables damage down and recycle additives of cells, making sure that your body commonly has amino acids, fatty acids, and one-of-a-kind constructing blocks. This recycling tool can be very essential for preserving cells running and making power while nutrients are scarce.

When cells are underneath lots of pressure, autophagy becomes a truthful greater crucial way to enhance their everyday normal performance. Whether the strain is because of changes inside the availability of nutrients, matters inside the environment, or a few element else, cells that undergo autophagy are better able to adjust and respond. Autophagy makes the surroundings indoors cells higher and greater inexperienced by using way of having rid of broken or vain factors.

Water fasting triggers autophagy, which makes cells more potent in methods that waft past honestly existence. It lets in the frame's contemporary health via making sure that the system internal cells works well, which facilitates vital duties like making electricity, managing indicators, and metabolic strategies.

In cease, the fact that autophagy permits cells work at their awesome for the duration of starvation suggests how bendy and self-shielding the frame is. This method no longer most effective continues cells operating after they have no outdoor vitamins, but it furthermore devices the body up to thrive with the useful resource of making cells more resilient, adaptable, and healthful generally whilst it's miles fasting.

Optimal Cellular Functioning

The capacity of the body to undergo model in response to numerous stressors is the purpose why right cellular function sooner or later of fasting is so essential. The manner of autophagy, it surely is initiated by means of manner of water fasting, functions as a mechanism that builds resistance. By eliminating defective mobile components, it gives an surroundings wherein cells are capable of reply efficiently to masses of stresses, which incorporates as shifts inside the availability of vitamins or problems posed with the resource of the environment. Because of their plasticity, cells are able to navigate and triumph over problems in a far higher and inexperienced manner, that's critical for the general properly-being of the organism.

Chapter 7: Combining Water Fasting With Other Lifestyles

When you integrate water fasting and exercise, you get a powerful balance that makes use of the great factors of every, supplying you with a more complete fitness and properly being plan. Fasting, a rustic wherein the body receives power from stored reserves, and exercise pass hand in hand, making a very unique putting for better fats usage and cell restore. The complicated way that fasting and exercise paintings collectively makes for a complete plan to beautify digestive and bodily fitness.

The benefits are:

Using fats

Ketosis Amplification: When you speedy, your frame is going into ketosis, a metabolic united states in which it uses saved fat for energy. This impact is more potent even as you exercising, specially aerobic obligations, even as you're fasting. The body gets better at burning fats quick, which enables with weight reduction and higher metabolic feature efficaciously.

Energy Use: When you rapid and workout session together, your frame learns to apply fat as a meals deliver first. This not best enables you shed kilos, but it additionally makes you more durable due to the fact your body learns a way to use its fat stores for lengthy-lasting electricity.

Better mobile repair: Exercise, in particular the type that makes you figure out, hastens autophagy, a manner in cells that receives rid of broken additives and recycles them. Fasting notably will growth autophagy, which has consequences that art work together to assist cells heal and renew themselves.

Cleaning and Rejuvenation: When you speedy and exercising at the identical time, autophagy starts going for walks, which begins offevolved a deep cleansing manner on your cells. This gets rid of components of cells that do not artwork proper and lets in make new, healthy cells, which is right for the fitness of cells as an entire.

Consideration:

Staying hydrated is important: To avoid becoming dehydrated, it is very essential to drink sufficient water on the same time as fasting and exercise. It is viable to lose greater fluids on the equal time as you speedy, and exercising ought to make this have an impact on worse. It's important to stay hydrated through ingesting water and, if crucial, electrolyte-wealthy drinks. This will help your body feature typically.

Electrolyte Balance: Electrolyte issues can take place on the equal time as you speedy for a long term or exercising consultation tough. Electrolyte-wealthy components or capsules help update misplaced minerals, which continues you from getting unwell from being dehydrated.

The Right Time:

Strategic Exercise Planning: Scheduling bodily activities for instances if you have extra energy, like right after a meal, can help you do higher and heal quicker. This planned time works with the body's herbal rhythms to make sure that exercise works well with fasting with out putting an excessive amount of stress on the body.

Balancing Intensity: It may be difficult to do immoderate-depth bodily sports at the identical time as fasting, particularly for lengthy quantities of time. Changing the sort and amount of depth of exercising based totally on everyone's electricity diploma is a long-time period and effective answer.

Helpful Hints for Integration:

Start Slowly: If you have got in no manner completed water fasting and workout collectively in advance than, begin with shorter fasting periods and sports which might be low to mild in energy. Let the body slowly get used to all of the stresses right away.

Pay interest on your frame: Watch out for signs and symptoms and signs and symptoms and symptoms of hunger, low electricity, and tiredness. Based on how the frame reacts to fasting, change how tough and the manner prolonged you discern out.

Include a Range of movements: Do a aggregate of aerobic, electricity education, and flexibility actions. This shape of bodily activities makes for a well-rounded health plan that works properly with fasting.

Post-Workout Nutrition: When you wreck your speedy after working out, devour ingredients which might be excessive in vitamins to help your frame heal and get greater power. Make superb you get the proper amount of right fats, carbohydrates, and proteins.

Working out and water fasting collectively have a strong impact that is going past the benefits of every one one after the other, offering an entire fitness answer. By cautiously combining those sports, human beings can take gain of the metabolic and cellular benefits, that could help them shed pounds and beautify their sizable health. When making any changes to your way of lifestyles, it is crucial to make certain that the plan fits your health, workout degree, and desires. Talking to scientific medical doctors or fitness professionals can give you custom designed advice to help you effectively and correctly comprise water fasting and exercising into your every day existence.

It is possible to attain your metabolic desires thru combining water fasting and the ketogenic weight loss program.

Working together, water fasting and the ketogenic food regimen are like powerful tools that work together to help your metabolism. While water fasting places your body right proper right into a state called ketosis, the ketogenic food regimen continues your frame in this country even while you're not fasting. The paintings together to make a sturdy environment for long-term fats metabolism, weight loss, and mind enhancements. This all-round technique is a one-of-a-kind way to enhance every highbrow and physical fitness.

Ketosis that lasts:

Rapid Induction of Ketosis: When you rapid on water, your body is going right into a nation called ketosis. In this united states, it stops the usage of glucose as fuel and starts using fat shops as an alternative. This first purpose while fasting gadgets the volume for ketosis to last for a long time.

Ketogenic Diet Maintenance: The ketogenic eating regimen maintains you in ketosis even at the same time as you are no longer fasting as it focuses on consuming few carbs and a number of fat. This combined effect creates a ordinary metabolic surroundings that enables burn fat, which leads to weight loss and a higher frame makeup.

Advantages for the mind:

Better Mental Clarity: Both the ketogenic food regimen and water fasting were associated with better highbrow clarity. Ketones are used as an possibility gasoline deliver inside the ketogenic weight loss plan, which allows maintain mind energy levels sturdy. Fasting moreover improves brain function.

Increased Cognitive Benefits: Doing each sports collectively may additionally moreover boom the cognitive advantages. Ketones live inside the body all through fasting and non-fasting times, which improves highbrow readability, reputation, and everyday mind characteristic.

Consideration

Adaptation over the years:

Transitioning Approach: To get the maximum out of the experience, it's miles quality to ease into every exercises over the years. Starting with shorter fasting home home windows lets in the body get used to going longer quantities of time without food, and easing into a ketogenic weight-reduction plan enables the frame get used to the change in macronutrient consumption.

Individualized Adaptation: The ketogenic weight loss program and fasting ought to have specific consequences on specific human beings. Gradual version helps you to tailor your treatment, reducing the threat of issue results and improving lengthy-time period compliance.

Foods High in Nutrients: Breaking the Fast Mindfully: It can be very critical to eat nutrient-dense, keto-first-class food at the same time as breaking a short, especially at the identical time as beginning a ketogenic food plan. This makes nice the body gets the vitamins it wishes while moreover supporting ketosis remaining.

Balanced Macronutrients: Eating meals with the right amount of carbs, proteins, and correct fat helps maintain your vitamins degree up. This is specifically crucial if you are on a ketogenic food regimen to make sure you do now not skip over out on any vitamins.

Helpful Hints for Integration

Focus on Hydration: It may be very vital to live sparkling even as fasting and on a ketogenic weight-reduction plan. Getting enough water lets in your metabolism and is ideal for your fashionable health.

Monitoring Electrolytes: Both of those items can exchange the stableness of electrolytes. Adding electrolyte-rich meals or vitamins to your healthy eating plan can help keep your body balanced, hold you hydrated, and reduce the chance of factor results.

Monitoring on a ordinary foundation: Regular check-u.S.With blood assessments can show how the frame is reacting to the combined technique. This we might also want to changes be made based totally on honestly everybody's fitness elements.

Mindful observation: It's crucial to be aware about how people react, how a tremendous deal power they've, and the manner they experience common. If you word adjustments within the fasting window, the meals you consume, or your famous method, you could make changes if you want to make the enjoy closing and be unique to you.

By walking together, water fasting and the ketogenic diet regime can help those who want to beautify their metabolic fitness. When executed slowly and with attention, this method has many advantages, from maintaining the fat metabolism going to improving mind function. Before making any adjustments to your way of lifestyles, you need to speak to a scientific physician or nutritionist to make certain that the new plan will assist you reach your fitness desires and conditions. Combining water fasting and the ketogenic food plan in a manner that works for you is an entire manner to enhance your metabolism and manual your bodily and highbrow fitness.

Finding Spiritual Balance in Water Fasting: Linking the Physical and the Divine

Water fasting is greater than honestly suitable on your health; it crosses over into the holy land of non secular and religious practices. When you combine fasting with religious practices, they artwork collectively in a powerful way to help you be healthful in each way, collectively with the spiritual and the physical. By searching into the hyperlink between water fasting and spirituality, we find out a manner to exercise electricity of will, area, and deep idea, connecting the bodily journey with a deep spiritual journey.

Advantages:

Reflection with Mind.

Prayerful Meditation: When you fast, you locate time for your self, pray, and meditate in a holy way. By deciding on not to devour or drink, humans can flip their attention inward, that can help them join deeply with their internal selves.

Higher Spiritual Awareness: Fasting places you in a quiet usa that makes it plenty less complicated to have a better spiritual cognizance. Although the frame is being cleansed, the mind is becoming extra in touch with the religious global.

Discipline and controlling yourself: Getting higher at situation: Spiritual rituals and fasting every in truth assist human beings grow to be more disciplined. Giving up meals on reason takes numerous power of will that is going beyond bodily energy of mind and into the arena of religious problem.

Helps with Personal Growth: Spiritual practices and fasting art work together to assist with every personal and non secular boom. The area you amplify on the same time as fasting goes past the bodily act itself. It impacts all components of your existence and makes you stronger.

Consideration

Setting the intention.

Aligning Physical and Spiritual Goals: Going into water fasting with a easy reason permits be a part of the physical act with religious desires. Setting clean dreams, prayers, or guarantees allows the quick gain non secular success thru giving it a beneficial framework.

Conscious hyperlink: Setting an purpose about fasting turns it from a physical exercising right right into a conscious link with God. The cause will become the compass that guides the adventure, whether or not it is to find out spiritual clarity, gratitude, or transcendence.

Respect for the beyond

Cultural and Religious Adherence: Following cultural and religious regulations in some unspecified time in the future of fasting instances makes sure that intellectual and physical practices pass hand in hand. Traditions which can be legit add a diploma of reverence to fasting and be part of humans to a bigger non secular enterprise.

Adding Sacred Rituals: Fasting turns into a sacred exercise on the same time as it is combined with rituals which can be required via one's faith or cultural customs. Rituals like set prayer instances and community get-togethers deliver the fasting duration a feel of holy cause.

When you combine spiritual practices with water fasting, you get a extra entire picture of health, in which the physical and the spiritual come together in a cute dance. This aggregate enables with deep non-public and religious increase. It can be finished through using fasting to assist with aware meditation, through the usage of going for walks towards self-control to collect project, or by the use of setting spiritual desires on motive.

Helpful Hints for Spiritual Integration:

Places of Worship: Set aside a place to need, meditate, or assume inside the path of the fasting time. People who workout spirituality can visit this holy area to be on my own.

Include Sacred Texts: During the fasting time, have a look at and reflect onconsideration on sacred texts or teachings. There is more non secular meaning on this, and it feeds the mind and soul.

Communal Connection: Take detail in religious sports activities sports with particular human beings, like virtual gatherings, shared prayers, or agency rituals. The spiritual journey is better even as people proportion research.

Gratitude Journaling: Write down spiritual insights, moments of connection, and expressions of gratitude in a gratitude pocket ebook at the equal time as you rapid. This practice of mirrored photo makes the non secular facet of fasting stronger.

When you rapid from water and do spiritual workout workouts at the equal time, they weave together to make a masterpiece that is going past the physical and into the divine. People who bypass in this two-element journey experience the advantages of highbrow boom, situation, and conscious mirrored image all at the equal time. This creates an entire-character technique to fitness that blessings the body, mind, and spirit. Always get assist from medical professionals and religious leaders to make certain that these practices fit your dreams and goals, for a balanced and pleasant revel in.

Chapter 8: Celebrating Wins A Motivational Boost

Celebrate small wins whilst you're fasting to shed pounds it will keep you going.

You want to be thrilled with yourself for starting to rapid that permits you to shed pounds. To stay induced and dedicated, you want to apprehend and characteristic a notable time small victories alongside the way. Recognizing your achievement, regardless of how small, is a powerful way to keep up the best changes you are making in your life?

What It Means: When you are attempting to shed pounds, gambling small wins technique more than surely searching at the numbers on the dimensions It method being privy to how your lifestyle, conduct, and thoughts-set are converting as a whole. In order to help you shed kilos, those small wins upload up and create a brilliant momentum that moves you forward.

Successfully Completing Fasts: It's a huge deal whilst you effectively surrender a fast, whether or not or now not it is a shorter bizarre fast or an extended one. When completed carefully and correctly, fasting let you shed pounds through leaving you with fewer strength than you want and inspiring your frame to use fats for strength. Celebrating the prevent of a short is a extraordinary manner to reveal that you are disciplined, strong, and committed to your weight reduction dreams.

Positive Lifestyle Changes: Making incredible adjustments on your existence is essential, even in case you're not fasting. Making changes like ingesting better, being greater lively, or choosing ingredients more cautiously may be examples of those adjustments. By noticing these modifications, you useful useful resource the concept that dropping weight isn't only a depend of brief-time period steps, but an prolonged-time period trade in the manner you stay your lifestyles.

Encouragement to Keep Going: Celebrating small wins is a superb way to preserve yourself advocated. Dopamine, the "experience-actual" neurotransmitter, is launched, which makes you experience real approximately the sports you take. This appropriate remarks makes you greater decided to preserve making healthful options, which enables your weight loss adventure remaining longer.

Getting More Confident: Every little win permits you enjoy more assured. As you be aware success, although it's first-rate a touch, you begin to receive as proper with that you could make changes at the manner to final. This developing self belief permits you live devoted for your weight loss goals and offers you the energy to stand demanding conditions with power and pressure.

How to Enjoy Small Victories.

Write them down in a magazine: Keep a diary to write down all of your accomplishments, irrespective of how small. In this elegance can be desirable fasts, extra active manner of lifestyles modifications, or better eating conduct.

Set Milestones: To assist you lose weight, set practical dreams for yourself. Enjoy meeting every goal, whether or not it's miles dropping a extremely good quantity of weight or sticking to a certain fasting agenda for a long time.

Treat Yourself: As a prize to your hard paintings, supply yourself something that isn't always food. This must suggest some aspect from getting a brand new outfit to performing some element amusing which you enjoy.

Share Your Success: Tell a friend, member of the family, or online organization in an effort to guide you approximately your successes. Sharing your accomplishments now not simplest makes you more devoted, however it also makes unique humans more likely that will help you.

Think About Your Progress: Take a moment to reflect onconsideration on how a long way you have got come. Take observe of the great modifications to your body, thoughts, and contemporary health. This perception is a robust motivation.

In the setting of fasting to shed pounds, celebrating small wins is an critical a part of an extended-time period and excessive exceptional journey. It turns the approach of dropping weight from a list of troubles to a list of successes, which makes the adventure extra amusing and motivating. Recognizing and praising your improvement will help you stay dedicated, maintain you stimulated, and set you up for extended-time period fulfillment for your weight loss dreams.

Chapter 9: What is water?

Water is a colorless and odorless substance found all over Earth. Water is made up of billions of molecules. Each molecule is made of one oxygen and two hydrogen atoms held together by strong covalent bonds.

Water is found in three different forms on Earth – gas, solid, and liquid. The form water takes depends on the temperature. Water on our planet flows as liquid in rivers, streams, and oceans; is solid as ice at the North and South Poles; and is gas (vapor) in the atmosphere. Water is also underground and inside plants and animals. All living things need water in some form to survive on Earth. People can go weeks without food, but can live only a few days without water.

Water is an important resource with many uses including food production, cleaning, transportation, power generation, recreation, and more.

Fifteen benefits of drinking water

Water is crucial for many bodily functions, such as lubricating the joints, delivering oxygen throughout the body, preventing kidney damage, and more.

Around 60 percent of the body is made up of water, and around 71 percent of the planet's surface is covered by water.

Perhaps it is the ubiquitous nature of water that means drinking enough each day is not at the top of many people's lists of priorities.

1. It lubricates the joints

Cartilage, found in joints and the disks of the spine, contains around 80 percent water. Long-term dehydration can reduce the joints' shock-absorbing ability, leading to joint pain.

2. It forms saliva and mucus

Saliva helps us digest our food and keeps the mouth, nose, and eyes moist. This prevents friction and damage. Drinking water also keeps the mouth clean. Consumed instead of sweetened beverages, it can also reduce tooth decay.

3. It delivers oxygen throughout the body

Blood is more than 90 percent water, and blood carries oxygen to different parts of the body.

4. It boosts skin health and beauty

With dehydration, the skin can become more vulnerable to skin disorders and premature wrinkling.

5. It cushions the brain, spinal cord, and other sensitive tissues

Dehydration can affect brain structure and function. It is also involved in the production of hormones and neurotransmitters. Prolonged dehydration can lead to problems with thinking and reasoning.

6. It regulates body temperature

Water that is stored in the middle layers of the skin comes to the skin's surface as sweat when the body heats up. As it evaporates, it cools the body. In sport.

Some scientists have suggested thatTrusted Source when there is too little water in the body, heat storage increases and the individual is less able to tolerate heat strain.

Having a lot of water in the body may reduce physical strain if heat stress occurs during exercise. However, more research is needed into these effects.

7, The digestive system depends on it

The bowel needs water to work properly. Dehydration can lead to digestive problems, constipation, and an overly acidic stomach. This increases the risk of heartburn and stomach ulcers.

8. It flushes body waste

Water is needed in the processes of sweating and removal of urine and feces.

9. It helps maintain blood pressure

A lack of water can cause blood to become thicker, increasing blood pressure.

10. The airways need it

When dehydrated, airways are restricted by the body in an effort to minimize water loss. This can make asthma and allergies worse.

11. It makes minerals and nutrients accessible

These dissolve in water, which makes it possible for them to reach different parts of the body.

12. It prevents kidney damage

The kidneys regulate fluid in the body. Insufficient water can lead to kidney stones and other problems.

13. It boosts performance during exercise

Dehydration during exercise may hinder performance.

Some scientists have proposed that consuming more water might enhance performance during strenuous activity.

More research is needed to confirm this, but one review found that dehydration reduces performance in activities lasting longer than 30 minutes.

14. Weight loss

Water may also help with weight loss, if it is consumed instead of sweetened juices and sodas. “Preloading” with water before meals can help prevent overeating by creating a sense of fullness.

15. It reduces the chance of a hangover

When partying, unsweetened soda water with ice and lemon alternated with alcoholic drinks can help prevent overconsumption of alcohol.

5 benefits of drinking water in the morning

Drinking water is very important for many bodily processes. These include transporting nutrients to cells, regulating the body’s temperature, and lubricating the joints.

If a person replaces their usual morning drink with water, it could provide them with several associated health benefits of increased water consumption.

1. For weight loss

Some people believe that drinking water in the morning can aid in weight loss.

For example, a 2019 studyTrusted Source found that higher fluid intake had links with improved body composition in young adults.

Before main meals, including breakfast

An older study from 2010Trusted Source found that middle-aged and older adults lost more weight when they drank 500 milliliters (ml) of water before each meal over 12 weeks.

Researchers partly attributed this weight loss to the decrease in energy intake from meals among the participants who drank water. This means they ate less food than individuals who did not partake in water before meals.

Thermogenesis

Thermogenesis is the production of heat. When a person drinks cold water, thermogenesis occurs to warm up the water entering the body, which burns calories.

An older study from 2013Trusted Source involved the water intake of 50 girls, with a body mass index of 25 to 29.9, along with a nutritious diet. It found that their body weight had decreased after they increased their water intake to 500 ml, three times a day, for 8 weeks. Participants drank the water before breakfast, lunch, and dinner.

Researchers attributed the weight loss to water-induced thermogenesis.

However, these studies cannot definitively claim that only the water intake led to the weight loss.

Additionally, the results do not necessarily mean that drinking water specifically in the morning offers weight loss effects.

2. For mental performance

Water can have an impact on cognition and mental performance — even minor dehydration can have adverse effects on cognition, according to a 2016 study.

A 2019 reviewTrusted Source looked at the effect of hydration on cognitive performance. It found that there was a trend of improved mental performance in hydrated study participants. However, the researchers noted that the results were not statistically significant.

Additionally, participants in the study drank water throughout the day. This may suggest that hydration throughout the day may be necessary for better mental performance rather than just drinking water in the morning.

Another 2019 studyTrusted Source on male college students found that dehydration had negative effects on short-term memory and attention. Short-term memory and attention improved once the participants rehydrated again.

Therefore, if a person wishes to increase their mental performance, specifically in the morning, drinking water may help.

3. Boosting mood

Drinking water may also have positive effects on a person’s mood.

A 2014 studyTrusted Source found that people who usually drank low volumes of water had better moods when they increased their water intake.

The same research found that when individuals — who normally drank high volumes of water — decreased their water intake, they experienced more thirst, decreased contentedness, and a reduction in calmness and positive emotions.

A 2019 studyTrusted Source also found that dehydration negatively affected mood, while rehydration improved mood and fatigue symptoms.

With this in mind, a person may wish to drink water throughout the whole day to experience prolonged positive effects on their mood.

4. For the skin

Some people believe that an increase in fluid intake can improve the appearance and health of the skin.

The skin contains about 30%Trusted Source water, which helps the skin remain plump, improving its elasticity and resilience.

An older study from 2015Trusted Source found that increased water intake may have a positive effect on skin physiology — it appeared more hydrated, especially in participants who usually drank less water.

A 2018 reviewTrusted Source found that increasing water intake may improve the hydration of the outer layer of the skin. However, the researchers noted that it was unclear whether this would benefit older adults.

However, even adequate skin hydration may not be sufficient to prevent wrinkles or offset the effects of the sun, genetics, or the environment.

Drinking water throughout the day may therefore help a person hydrate their skin, but they may not notice significant changes in its appearance.

5. For other bodily functions

Adequate water intake is also important in many body functions.

Kidneys: Drinking water can help the kidneys remove wastewater from the body.

Urinary tract: According to an older studyTrusted Source from 2010, increased fluid intake may prevent urolithiasis, which occurs when stones are present in the urinary tract.

Cardiovascular system: A 2019 studyTrusted Source found that people require adequate water intake for proper cardiovascular system function. The study noted that dehydration and inadequate water intake negatively affected blood pressure regulation and vascular function.

Joints and bones: Water is a component of the lubricating fluid around the joints, which could help relieve joint pain.

Risks

Some potential risks of drinking water in the morning may involve:

Drinking too much: If a person drinks too much water, water toxicityTrusted Source can occur. This can have negative effects on brain function, including confusion, nausea, and vomiting.

Only drinking in the morning: If a person's water intake only occurs in the morning, there may be a risk that they are not meeting their optimal water intake, which can lead to dehydrationTrusted Source. Dehydration can lead to low mood and reduced cognition.

Drinking flavored water: A person may also rely too heavily on sugared drinks to meet their daily water intake. For example, flavored water and sweetened beverages contain more calories than plain water. A 2016 studyTrusted Source found that people who drank more plain water were more likely to lose weight and consume fewer calories. However, individuals could instead drink fruit or herb-infused flavored water or sparkling water.

Chapter 10: What Is Water Fasting?

Water fasting is solely consuming water, without any food at all, for the duration of the diet. It can be done for wellness reasons, or for religious and spiritual reasons. Water fasting should be approached with caution. While it may help you lose weight in the short term, water fasting is not a sustainable approach to weight loss and puts you at risk for certain health complications.

There are many different fasts and "detox diets" that promise to cleanse the body of toxins, promote weight loss, and improve health. But there is little scientific evidence to prove these diets—including water fasting—actually detoxify the body and support weight management.

There are some limited potential benefits to medically supervised water fasting diets, but most experts agree that the potential risks, particularly when attempted at home, far outweigh the benefits, and people with certain medical conditions should not attempt to water fast.

What You Can Eat

You can only drink water for the duration of the fast. Some studies that have been performed have participants drink mineral water so that at least some essential minerals could be absorbed during the fasting period.

What You Cannot Eat

A water fast is true to its name: It's a fast during which all food and drink except water are restricted. That means no coffee, no tea, no alcohol, no zero-calorie sports drinks, or any other beverage. This also means no food.

How to Prepare a Water Fast & Tips

Water fasts typically last 24 to 72 hours, but medically supervised water fasts may last longer.3 For your safety, you should not try to fast without medical clearance and supervision.

Because it is not a practice that is widely endorsed by the mainstream medical or nutritional community, there are no uniform guidelines for water fasting. Most of the available tips and practices come from first-person accounts of fasts shared by advocates without any medical or nutritional credentials.

There are a limited number of alternative medicine clinics that offer supervised water fasts. Many who undergo water fasting in a clinic environment begin the process with a referral from their healthcare provider.

Though water fasting is simple, that doesn't mean it's easy or safe.

In a clinical environment, patients are monitored regularly for signs of distress such as a foul taste in the mouth, lower back pain, skin rashes, discharges from mucous membranes, headaches, irritability, nausea, or vomiting. Regular blood and urine tests are also performed.

Many who perform water fasts at home do so without professional support and without the safety net provided by medical supervision. Because it is a fairly straightforward process, people may follow instructions found online or in magazines.

Though water fasting is simple, that doesn't mean it's easy or safe. During a fast, you can't consume anything but water. You generally drink at least 2 to 3 liters of water per day (ideally water consumption would be at the higher end of that range because you will not get the water you normally get from food).

Water fasting is harmful but can be especially detrimental to people with certain medical conditions. Never try a water fast if you have any of these conditions.

Chronic kidney disease: Fasting may worsen kidney function.

Diabetes: Fasting may increase the risk of diabetic ketoacidosis and hypoglycemia (low blood sugar).

Eating disorders: Fasting may lead to disordered eating patterns like a binge-restrict cycle.

Heartburn or gastroesophageal reflux disorder (GERD): Your stomach may continue to make stomach acid even without food, which can worsen symptoms of heartburn and GERD.

People who are pregnant or breastfeeding and children and teens under the age of 18 should also not water fast. Additionally, if you are a smoker, managing an addiction, or regularly take a prescription or over-the-counter medication, seek the personalized advice of your healthcare provider before fasting.

Pros of Water Fasting

There are possible benefits of water fasting, but it's important to note that research on the safety of a water fast is lacking, with substantial evidence pointing instead toward the potential risks.

Reduces alcohol, sugar, and sodium intake:

It is unclear whether or not the fasting procedure itself can lead to positive outcomes. For example, simply reducing your sugar or sodium intake for a few days may provide a benefit. And for those who drink regularly, avoiding alcohol for several days or more may lead to a reduction in blood pressure even with no other diet changes.

Lowers blood pressure:

Drinking more water and consuming less salt are two things associated with lower blood pressure readings. A water fast will enable you to do both of these things, which could help manage blood pressure. Medically supervised water fasts have shown to be effective in lowering blood pressure in patients with borderline hypertension.

Promotes cell recycling:

Every day, your cells are broken down and recycled. This process is called autophagy, and it's thought that it may play a role in preventing cancer, heart disease, and Alzheimer's disease.Unfortunately, the research on the relationship between water fasting and autophagy in humans is far too limited to know for sure.

Lowers risk of heart disease:

There is limited evidence that water fasting can help with heart disease. One study enrolled 30 apparently healthy volunteers into a 24-hour water fast. At the end of the fast, the participants showed lower levels of triglycerides and cholesterol, two big risk factors for cardiovascular disease.

Helps protect against diabetes:

Research shows that fasting of any type may help to improve insulin sensitivity. Insulin resistance is the main factor in the development of type 2 diabetes, so it's possible that short water fasts can improve insulin sensitivity and decrease the risk of diabetes.

Cons of Water Fasting

While there may be some health advantages of fasting with water, there are also significant risks and drawbacks.

Digestive upset:

After restricting calories for an extended period, consuming food again (especially in larger amounts) can cause digestive discomfort and nausea.

Risk of refeeding syndrome:

Though unlikely, people who reintroduce calories too quickly after extended fasting are at higher risk for refeeding syndrome, a potentially fatal condition that involves rapid metabolic changes, usually in people who are extremely malnourished.Refeeding syndrome is most often a consideration in those living with eating disorders. In clinical settings, some guidelines suggest that calories be reintroduced very slowly (using nutritional supplements and increasing by only 10 to 30 calories per day) to avoid refeeding syndrome.

May cause nutrient deficiencies:

Any fasting protocol can put you at risk for nutrient deficiencies. By restricting calories, you also limit your intake of essential vitamins, minerals, fatty acids, amino acids, and electrolytes—all things your body needs to function correctly.

May cause dehydration:

Even though you drink water during a water fast, you can be at risk for dehydration. For most people, at least 20% of daily water consumption comes from the foods you eat. If you don't increase your water intake during the fast, you will consume much less water than usual.

Unsafe blood pressure changes:

If you drink too much water, you may experience hypotension. Hypotension is extremely low blood pressure—the opposite of hypertension, or high blood pressure. Additionally, you may experience orthostatic hypotension, which involves sudden drops in blood pressure upon standing up. Orthostatic hypotension can cause dizziness and lightheadedness.

Hyponatremia:

Also called water intoxication, hyponatremia occurs when the water and salt lost through sweating are replaced by water only. You shouldn't exercise during a water fast because you lose salt through perspiration and won't replace it by eating food or drinking sports beverages.

Unable to be physically active:

In addition to the dangers of hyponatremia, it is difficult to be physically active, a vital aspect of health, because this diet contributes to lack of energy. Some studies have demonstrated that fasting causes decreased performance across a range of different fitness activities.

Dizziness, fatigue, and trouble focusing:

Dizziness, fatigue, and brain fog are all symptoms of extreme calorie restriction. Researchers have found that even in healthy young women, balance and stability control may be compromised during fasting.When you don't consume the number of calories your body needs, your body will struggle to perform at an optimal level. It may become difficult to focus at work or school during a water fast. Fasting can also cause mild to severe headaches.

May lead to binge eating:

Fasting—and dieting or restricting calories in general—often leads to binge eating.16 Fasting can also lead to obsessive or intrusive thoughts about food, which may cause you to binge eat when your water fast is over.

To achieve many, if not all, of the purported health benefits of a water fast, there are often safer, healthier approaches. For example, you might try reducing your sodium or alcohol intake as part of a healthy diet instead.

Is Water Fasting a Healthy Choice for You?

The 2020-2025 USDA Dietary Guidelines offer recommendations and tips for a balanced diet, which should include a variety of vegetables, fruits, grains, lean meats, beans, legumes, nuts, seeds, dairy, and healthy oils.

The water fast excludes all of these healthy food groups, so it does not adhere to USDA guidelines and is therefore not considered a healthy way to lose weight. As a short-term diet, you may see some weight loss during a water fast, but only for a few days. When you restrict your caloric intake for 24 hours or more, you may notice a temporary reduction in weight that lasts for a few days, which is the result of water weight and glycogen, not necessarily actual fat loss or a lasting change in your body mass.

Keep in mind that this weight loss is probably in the form of water weight and glycogen (stored carbohydrates), and not actual fat loss. It takes a few days for your body to begin burning stored fat because it uses available energy like glucose and glycogen first.

A healthy diet and regular exercise are integral to successful long-term weight loss. Use the following tool to calculate how many calories you should consume each day to reach your weight loss goals.

Due to the restrictive nature of water fasting, this diet does not adhere to USDA guidelines and is not considered a healthy way to lose weight. Rapid weight loss in the form of water weight is not sustainable for long-term weight management.

Chapter 11: 7 day water fast before and after

If you were to take a before and after picture of your 7-day water fast then you'll find you lost at least 10 pounds.

Most people who do a 7-day water fast end up losing anywhere from 10-20 pounds after the week is up.

A lot of it depends on how much weight you have to lose in the first place, where you currently are with your health and other factors such as the efficiency of your metabolism.

But consider the average 7-day weekly weight loss is 1-2 pounds. So you'll be getting a 5-10x more weight loss than the norm.

7 day water fast benefits

There are more than a handful of benefits to doing a 7-day water fast other than weight loss.

This study alone found fasting was effective for losing weight, lowering blood pressure and reducing oxidative stress.

The fasting process has been found to promote autophagy. This is your body's process of killing off dangerous cancerous cells in the body.

Studies have also found fasting helps to regenerate stem cells. As the years go by your body becomes less and less efficient and stem cell regeneration.

Since you won't have any food coming in you can expect for your insulin sensitivity to improve. This is great to help reduce your risk of diabetes which in itself can cause weight gain.

You'll lower the inflammation in your body while fasting for 7 days. This, in turn, will help your body repair and heal as well as fighting the aging process.

Studies have found fasting helps to lower the risk of heart disease too. If you have any symptoms or wish to better prevent heart disease then it's a good idea to consider fasting.

You can also expect gut health problems to improve as well. This will give your gut time to heal and recover since it won't have any food to process for a while.

The health of your skin will also improve with stem cell regeneration and less inflammation. If you have any skin conditions or wish to improve its appearance then fasting can help.

Heart disease is the biggest killer in the world today. Fasting has been found to lower the risk of heart disease.

Some other extra benefits include realizing what hunger really means. Just because you feel hungry doesn't mean you always have to go to the kitchen and scarf down. If you know these feelings of hunger will pass then you'll be less likely to overeat down the road.

Plus you'll get a greater sense of control over your future thoughts. You'll have more power of those uncontrollable feelings of hunger after making it through the 7-day fast.

7 Day Water Fasting Dangers

Now that you know the amazing benefits that come from a 7-day water fast you should also know about the dangers.

If you don't have any health issues then for the majority of people doing a 7-day water fast will be completely fine. Other than periods of hunger you should actually end up better off after the fast than you were before it.

But if you have any medical issues then it's a wise and recommended idea to first talk to your doctor. Or if you have or have had an eating disorder in the past then this might not be the best for you.

Some common medical reasons for not doing a 7-day water fast include hypoglycemia, taking medications, recent surgeries, and if you are pregnant/nursing.

And try to use your common sense and monitor yourself during your fast. If you feel anything is off during the 7 days while fasting then it'll be a wise idea to stop.

Water Fasting Hacks

It doesn't take a rocket scientist to know not eating anything for 7 days is going to be tough at times.

That's why I wanted to share with you some of these tips you can use to better improve the odds you successfully complete a 7-day water fast.

If people are constantly eating right in front of you then it's going to be that much harder to stick to the fast. I'd even go so far as to stay away walking by restaurants and the grocery store. The fewer temptations the better.

Since this is a water fast it's critical to make sure you drink lots and lots of water. It'll not only keep you hydrated but it'll also help to fill out your stomach. This will help to lessen the feelings of hunger.

If you ever find yourself feeling woozy and your muscles cramping then start taking some electrolytes. You can add a small pinch of Himalayan pink salt to a glass of water to help too.

What Happens to Your Body During a 7 Day Water Fast

Day 1:

If you've done Intermittent Fasting for weight loss before then this won't be too difficult. There will be small waves of hunger earlier in the day. As the day goes on your body is so used to food you'll get some hunger pangs. Expect to maybe have feelings of irritability in the afternoon but it's usually nothing unbearable. This is when your mental toughness will be needed to kick this 7-day water fast for weight loss off successfully.

Day 2-3:

You'll probably wake up feeling ok in the morning but don't be surprised if you crash hard not much longer after. The majority of people say Days 2-3 are going to be the toughest to get through. You'll feel the most hunger during these first few days. Just remember to keep motivated and hang in there. The feelings of being bloated will start to go away and your body will begin to feel lighter. Don't worry if you get a little brain fog too it's your body dumping all the toxins out of the system as autophagy kicks in.

Day 4:

This is when the energy levels should really start coming back to you. Your body begins to realize what's going on and will start using your fat stores for energy. After you get over that first 3 days you'll experience a sense of empowerment. You'll begin waking up feeling good once again and can start getting more stuff done. Expect much of the brain fog to go away and you'll have more mental clarity.

Day 5-7:

You'll continue to wake up with much better energy than those first few days. Your body is no longer working to digest foods while you sleep so you should be feeling a lot better. You'll still have experiences with hunger but it's usually nothing crazy like before. Many people have ups and downs during these last few days but overall actually feel quite good. As the 7-day water fast comes to a close you'll feel like you're on cloud nine as you just successfully completing a 7-day water fast.

How Much Weight Can You Lose if You Fast for One Week?

Most people report losing anywhere from 10-20 pounds while on a 7-day water fast. This is a big number compared to the average weight loss of 1-2 pounds per week. Just keep in mind you'll also be losing muscle, water & glycogen stores while fasting too. It's not all from fat.

Can You Lose 10 Pounds in a Week?

Yes, it's definitely possible with a water fast. It's not something you're going to want to do often but most people report on the lesser side losing 10 pounds in a week. At the top range you can expect to lose up to 20 pounds in the week. You can lose 20 pounds in 2 weeks with less intense methods too.

50 Best Detox Waters for Fat Burning and Weight Loss

1 GRAPEFRUIT/MINT

Aside from being as refreshingly tart as an Amy Schumer routine, grapefruit has serious health benefits: A study published in the journal Metabolism found that those who ate grapefruit for six weeks lost a full inch off their waistlines. Why? The fruit is rich in phytochemicals, a bioactive compound that burns fat. And mint has been known to suppress appetite. One study published in the Journal of Neurological and Orthopaedic Medicine found that people who sniffed peppermint every two hours lost an average of 5 pounds a month!

2 BLUEBERRY/LEMONADE

Skip the sugary, syrupy soft-drink version and go for cleansing freshness at a fraction of the calories. Drop in a few sprigs of mint for a natural appetite suppressant.

3 APPLE/LEMON/MINT

Lemon is a common detox ingredient for good reason: An antioxidant in its peel stimulates liver enzymes to help flush toxins from the body. Here, it's paired with apple, one of our best fruits for a better body!

4 RASPBERRY/LEMON

The last time you saw this flavor combo, it was probably on a menu describing a super-caloric iced tea. Forget that and make this version, which will be refreshing and energizing without a sugar crash.

5 ORANGE/LEMON/LIME

Three citrus fruits work together in this cleansing detox water: All three are rich in D-limonene, which has been shown to have anti-cancer effects and soothe heartburn and acid reflux. It also flushes toxins and helps clear up irregularity.

6 MINT/MELON

Stock up on the last of the summer watermelon while you can: It's one of the very best fruits for fat loss, having been shown to improve lipid (fat) profiles and decrease the accumulation of body fat.

What's more, a Spanish study found that athletes who drank watermelon juice post-workout had less muscle soreness.

7 CUCUMBER/LIME/KIWI

Cucumbers are a known diet staple, and for good reason: they're extremely low in calories, and their skin contains tons of vitamins and minerals for your body to benefit from. So when adding to your H2O, be sure to keep the skin on.

8 FIG/STRAWBERRY

This water may not help you get ripped, but the nutrients figs contain, including potassium, help your muscles work. They're also a great source of fiber, which will help slow digestion and keep you feeling fuller, longer.

9 ORANGE/LEMON/MINT

Citrus fruits are classic ingredients: They're rich in the antioxidant D-limonene, a powerful compound found in the peel that stimulates liver enzymes to help flush toxins from the body and gives sluggish bowels a kick, according to the World Health

Organization. Drinking several glasses of citrusy water daily can help you lose belly fat.

10 ORANGE/POMEGRANATE/CINNAMON

Cinnamon is a great way to add some sweetness to your drink without the excess calories as other sugary additives would. Pomegranates are also a great addition for an antioxidant boost, and oranges are filled with essential vitamins and minerals to keep your body slim and healthy.

11 BLACKBERRY/MINT

Blackberries are an amazing source for detox-boosting antioxidants. Adding mint to this fruit water will help give it a refreshing taste while promoting digestion and soothing your indigestion and inflammation.

12 LEMON/CELERY/CUCUMBER

Add celery to any water and crunch away! It has six calories per stalk and full of vitamins A, C, and K, as well as B vitamins (such as folate) and potassium, which diminishes water retention and aids muscle recovery, so you can get back in the gym sooner and burn more calories.

13 KIWI/CUCUMBER/MINT

This refreshing green detox water contains a secret superhero: Kiwi has been shown to reduce bloating and constipation and improve immunity. Cucumber is not only refreshing, but it's also high in vitamins C and K, so eat the veggie once you drain your glass.

14 POMEGRANATE/STRAWBERRY/MINT

Pomegranates are the stuff of ancient legend, and for good reason: The seeds have three kinds of antioxidant polyphenols, including tannins, anthocyanins, and ellagic acid, which all help fight and prevent damage to your body caused by free radicals.

15 FROZEN BERRY AND LEMON

Dropping berries into your glass is an excellent idea. Be they strawberries, blueberries, or blackberries, they're some of the best fat-burning foods. Using frozen berries gives your sip a pleasing mocktail effect.

16 MINT/ROSEMARY/LEMON/CUCUMBER

A blend of savory and sweet, this glass is good for staving off the munchies: Lemon and mint are natural appetite suppressants.

17 COCONUT/PERSIMMON

This one's a great option for detoxing after a gluttonous meal: Persimmons are rich in toxin-mopping vitamins A and C and high in, ahem, elimination-speeding fiber. They also have a small amount of manganese, which is important in the metabolism of fats and protein.

18 STRAWBERRY/ORANGE

strawberries cutting board

Shutterstock

Fat-burning berries plus body-cleansing lemon makes this detox water a total treat. Add some seltzer if you like, to bring back childhood Fanta memories absolutely guilt-free.

19 BERRY/KIWI/ORANGE

Berries are an excellent addition to your detox drinks since they're packed with antioxidants. But that's not the only nutritional star in this detox drink: oranges are filled with vitamin C to give you a boost of energy, and kiwis have tons of nutrients, like potassium, that are beneficial for weight loss.

20 RASPBERRY/BLUEBERRY/MINT

21 DRAGON FRUIT

Dragon fruit is not only tasty, but it also contains vital antioxidants and good fatty acids to help keep your body in tip-top shape. Bonus: it contains a hefty serving of calcium, iron, and lycopene, an inflammation-fighting antioxidant.

22 KIWI/WATERMELON

On top of being extremely refreshing, watermelon is one of the healthiest foods on the planet. That's because there are science-backed benefits: the University of Kentucky found that this fruit can help lower fat accumulation, and the Universidad Politécnica de Cartagena in Spain showed that watermelon actually helps reduce muscle soreness so you can make your gym session last a little longer.

23 LIME/CHIA

Lime is a soothing, cleansing veteran, but chia seeds are the hot upstarts of detox: They can stabilize blood sugar, boost weight loss, keep your hunger at bay and even help keep your body hydrated throughout the day: They expand to as much as 10 times their size when in liquid, helping you feel full and reducing your appetite!

24STRAWBERRY/CUCUMBER/PINEAPPLE

This detox water concoction is an inflammation-fighting powerhouse: pineapple and strawberries both have antioxidant properties. Cucumber is a low-cal and refreshing additive that is high in vitamins C and K.

25 KIWI/LEMON/PEAR

We all know that kiwis and limes are great to add into your detox diet, but what about pears? They're a great choice at only 100 calories and taste refreshing, too. Make sure you eat the pears after you take them out of your water; pears are chock-full of fiber that will keep you feeling fuller, longer.

26 STRAWBERRY/MINT/LEMON

This is a spa combo that not only tastes delicious but can also help reduce belly bloat: lemon is a natural diuretic, strawberry has antioxidants, and mint reduces appetite. Take this as a cue to experiment with flavors of your own.

27 LEMON/STRAWBERRY/CHIA

Strawberries are one of the best low-carb fruits to help you shed some pounds. They only contain 12 grams of carbs and possess natural chemicals called polyphenols that can actually stop fat cells from forming.

28 MANGO/GINGER

This detox water is a powerful bloat-fighter, thanks to fresh ginger. Used for thousands of years to ease queasy tummies and aid digestion, you'll find mentions of ginger in Chinese medical texts from the fourth century BC! Ginger acts as a muscle relaxant that allows the body to more easily expel gas, according to Herbal Medicine:

Biomolecular and Clinical Aspects. You can get your ginger fix in a variety of forms, though fresh ginger is richest in gingerol—the compound that contributes to many of the spice's health benefits.

29 GRAPEFRUIT/LEMON

Forget chemical-laden Fresca. Pour plain seltzer over fresh grapefruit and lemon for an energizing, fat-burning elixir.

30 GOJI/CUCUMBER/MINT

Goji berries add more than a sweet-and-tangy taste to your water: The superfood has a slimming effect! In a study published in the Journal of the American College of Nutrition, participants were either given a single dose of L. barbarum, the plant from which goji berries are harvested, or a placebo after a meal. The researchers found that one hour after the dose, the goji group was burning calories at a rate 10 percent higher than the placebo group. The effects lasted up to 4 hours! (Just be wary of any unwanted side effects: The energizing fruits are known as "the Viagra of China.")

31 POMEGRANATE

Throw away that sugary pomegranate juice cocktail and try this sweet detox drink instead. This detox water has all of the vitamins and nutrients that the fruit can supply, without all of the excess sugar and sweeteners.

32 CARROT/PERSIMMON

Now here's an orange drink worth downing by the bottle. Carrots are spiked with carotenoids—fat-soluble compounds that are associated with a reduction in a wide range of cancers, as well as reduced risk and severity of inflammatory conditions such as asthma and rheumatoid arthritis. Persimmons are rich in vitamins A, C and the antioxidant lycopene, an antioxidant which may reduce the risk of cancer.

33 RASPBERRY/STRAWBERRY

Talk about your double dose of berries: both strawberries and raspberries are great sources of fiber. This detox elixir will keep your digestive system working smoothly, so drink up and be sure to eat the fruit when you're done!

34 CRANBERRY/LEMON

Cranberries contain tons of fiber and also supply a hefty dose of vitamin C. According to the University of Maryland Medical Center, vitamin C is one of the most important antioxidants for removing damage-causing free radicals in your body and fighting against infectious diseases.

35 BLOOD ORANGE/GRAPE/MINT

For such a sweet fruit, blood oranges are actually pretty low in the calorie department at only 70 calories per serving, and they contain fiber and potassium. Grapes are also a great addition to your detox water since they have a high water content to keep you extra hydrated throughout your day.

36 CRANBERRY/PEACH/BLUEBERRY

Peaches are much more than just a sweet treat; they're a nutritional powerhouse for warding off obesity and the health risks that go with it. According to a study from the Texas A&M University, peaches and other stone fruits (like plums and nectarines) can lower your risk of excessive weight gain, diabetes, and cardiovascular disease.

37 APPLE/CINNAMON

Who knew apple cinnamon could work as well in water as it does in oatmeal? It's a good thing: Cinnamon balances blood sugar and wards off insulin spikes, which protects you from the munchies.

38 LEMON/APPLE/FIG

We all know that an apple a day keeps the doctor away, but what about figs? This exotic fruit is extremely high in fiber, a diet essential, and contains potassium to help lower blood pressure.

39 APPLE/MANDARIN/MINT/CHIA

Don't leave mandarin oranges to your aunt's Waldorf Salad. Two Japanese studies showed that drinking mandarin orange juice reduced participants' incidence of liver cancer. It's theorized that's due to oranges' high level of carotenoids, the pigment that gives the fruit its color and functions as a potent antioxidant, mopping up free radicals and repairing DNA damage that can cause disease.

40 BANANA/LEMON/MANGO/TOMATO

It may look unlikely, but this is a brilliant combo: Bananas are a good source of prebiotic fiber, which helps feed good gut bacteria and improve digestion; lemon cleanses the body; mangoes are packed with vitamin C, and tomatoes have cancer-fighting antioxidants. Just don't forget to snack on the slices.

41STRAWBERRY/PEAR/BLUEBERRY/KIWI

The tropical backdrop isn't the only thing we love about this one: Aside from fat-burning berries and bloat-fighting kiwi, pears contain catechins, antioxidants that hinder the storage of belly fat!

42 MELON/BLACKBERRY/ROSEMARY

You'll definitely want to guzzle down a bottle (or three) of this detox water: blackberries are known for their high antioxidant content, and melons promote a healthy digestive system through their high amounts of fiber. Rosemary is also a great source of antioxidants to keep your body on track to a healthier you.

43 WATERMELON/LEMON

Here's your new sports drink: Watermelon is rich in L-citrulline, an amino acid that helps move lactic acid out of muscles, reducing pain and fatigue. Lemon's appetite-suppressing effects will prevent you from ordering that cheeseburger you think you deserve.

44 WATERMELON WITH ALOE VERA

One of the great weight-loss secrets, aloe vera juice has been a mainstay in Ayurvedic medicine for centuries. The juice can help balance your digestive system, which will lessen belly bloat and keep things, um, moving.

45 DOUBLE BERRY/BASIL

Basil in your drink may seem odd at first, but it's actually refreshingly tasty. But that's not the only reason why this detox drink is on this list: basil is actually a known anti-inflammatory, which will get rid of all your bloating and discomfort in no time.

46 LEMON/CUCUMBER/MINT

Blast your muffin top away with this fruity elixir. The combination of lemon's abundant vitamin content, cucumber's high water retention, and mint's digestion-promoting powers will flatten your belly and keep you satisfied.

47 THREE BERRY LEMON

You've heard of the Wonder Twins? This has the Wonder Quadruplets. As mentioned, the polyphenols in berries torch flab (and even stop its formation before it starts!), and the powerful amino acids in lemon detoxify the liver and speed wastes out of the body (the old-fashioned way).

48 PINEAPPLE

They don't get much simpler than this water, and we love that. We also love that it has the sweetness of a tropical cocktail at a fraction of the calories, and that pineapple is loaded with bromelain, an enzyme that quells inflammation throughout the body (i.e. bloat, flab, and aching muscles).

49 APPLE/LEMON

We'd happily sip from this antioxidant-packed pitcher. Apples are one of the best fat-burning fruits; leave the peels on and snack away once you've drained your glass.

50 CUCUMBER/MINT/GINGER/CINNAMON

Ginger is definitely a detox ingredient you don't want to skip. It's a health powerhouse: it fights inflammation, treats chronic indigestion, and lowers blood sugar significantly, according to a 2015 study in the Iranian Journal of Pharmaceutical Research. It's no wonder it hails as one of the healthiest spices on the planet.

Chapter 9: Recipes

Jumbo prawns with tomatoes and garlic

Preparation time less than 30 mins

Cooking time less than 10 mins

Ingredients

1 tbsp mild olive oil

2 garlic cloves, very thinly sliced

1 long red chilli, deseeded and finely chopped (or use ½ tsp dried chilli flakes)

150g/5½oz cherry tomatoes, halved

½ lemon, juice only

250g/9oz jumbo king prawns, cooked, peeled and deveined

3 heaped tbsp roughly chopped flat leaf parsley

ground black pepper

160g/6oz green beans, steamed, to serve

Method

Heat the oil in a small frying pan over a low heat. Add the garlic and chilli and cook very gently for five minutes or until the garlic is very soft but not coloured, stirring occasionally.

Add the tomatoes and lemon juice and cook for two minutes or until beginning to soften. Stir in the prawns and cook for 2-3 minutes, stirring, until the tomatoes are well softened and the prawns are hot through.

Remove the pan from the heat, stir in the parsley, season with lots of pepper and serve with the beans.

Poached eggs with bacon and tomatoes

Preparation time less than 30 mins

Cooking time less than 10 mins

Ingredients

2 large ripe tomatoes, halved

4 rashers smoked back bacon, all visible fat removed

2 medium free-range eggs

ground black pepper

Method

Preheat the grill to its hottest setting. Put the tomatoes on a rack over a grill pan lined with foil. Season with pepper.

Grill for 3 minutes, then add the bacon and grill for a further 4 minutes, turning the bacon after 2 minutes so that it is lightly browned on both sides.

Meanwhile, half-fill a medium pan with water and bring it to the boil. Crack the eggs into two small bowls. Turn the heat down so that the water is bubbling very gently. Slowly add the eggs to the water and cook for 3 minutes or until the white is set but the yolk remains runny.

Using a slotted spoon, scoop the eggs out of the water and divide between two plates. Add the cooked bacon and tomatoes. Season with a little salt and pepper and serve.

Italian style meatballs with courgette 'tagliatelle'

Preparation time less than 30 mins

Cooking time 10 to 30 mins

Ingredients

For the meatballs

250g/9oz extra lean beef mince (5% fat or less)

1 small onion, very finely chopped

1 tsp dried mixed herbs

calorie controlled cooking oil spray

1 garlic clove, crushed

227g/8oz can chopped tomatoes

2 heaped tbsp finely shredded fresh basil leaves, plus extra to garnish

For the courgette 'tagliatelle'

2 medium courgettes, trimmed and deseeded

sea salt and freshly ground black pepper

Method

Place the beef, half the onion, half the mixed herbs and a pinch of salt and pepper in a bowl and mix well. Form into 10 small balls.

Spray a medium non-stick frying pan with a little oil and cook the meatballs for 5-7 minutes, turning occasionally until browned on all sides. Transfer to a plate.

For the sauce, put the remaining onion in the same pan and cook over a low heat for three minutes, stirring. Add the garlic and cook for a few seconds.

Stir in the tomatoes, 300ml/10fl oz water, the remaining mixed herbs and shredded basil. Bring to the boil, stirring. Return the meatballs to the pan, reduce the heat to a simmer and cook for 20 minutes, stirring occasionally until the sauce is thick and the meatballs are cooked throughout.

Meanwhile , half-fill a medium pan with water and bring to the boil. Use a vegetable peeler to peel the courgettes into ribbons. Cook the courgette in the boiling water for one minute then drain.

Divide the courgette ribbons between two plates and top with the meatballs and sauce. Garnish with basil leaves.

Crunchy banana yoghurt

Preparation time less than 30 mins

Cooking time no cooking required

Ingredients

340g/12oz fat-free natural Greek-style yoghurt

1 banana, peeled and sliced

15g/½oz mixed seeds (pumpkin, sesame and sunflower) (or use toasted flaked almonds)

Method

Divide the yoghurt between two small bowls. Scatter the banana on top.

Sprinkle with seeds or nuts and serve.

Chicken and vegetable balti

Preparation time less than 30 mins

Cooking time 30 mins to 1 hour

Ingredients

calorie controlled cooking oil spray

1 medium onion, thinly sliced

4 chicken thighs, boned and skinned

1 red pepper, deseeded and cut into 3cm/1in chunks

1 yellow pepper, deseeded and cut into 3cm/1in chunks

1 tbsp cornflour

150g/5½oz fat-free natural yogurt

1 tbsp medium or mild curry powder

2 garlic cloves, thinly sliced

227g/8oz tin chopped tomatoes

3 heaped tbsp finely chopped fresh coriander, plus extra to garnish

freshly ground black pepper

Method

Spray a large, deep, non-stick frying pan or wok with oil and place over a medium heat. Add the onion and cook for five minutes, stirring regularly until well softened and lightly browned.

Meanwhile, trim all the visible fat off the chicken thighs, cut each one into four pieces and season with black pepper.

Add the chicken and peppers into the pan with the onion and cook for three minutes, turning occasionally.

Meanwhile, in a small bowl, mix the cornflour with 2 tablespoons cold water and stir in the yoghurt until thoroughly mixed.

Sprinkle the curry powder over the chicken and vegetables, add the garlic and cook for 30 seconds.

Tip the tomatoes into the pan, add the yoghurt mixture, 150ml/3½fl oz of water and coriander.

Bring to a gentle simmer and cook for 20-25 minutes, stirring occasionally until the chicken is tender and the sauce is thick. Season with freshly ground black pepper to taste and garnish with coriander.

Berry yoghurt

Preparation time less than 30 mins

Cooking time no cooking required

Ingredients

175g/6oz frozen mixed berries, defrosted

340g/12oz fat-free Greek yoghurt

10g/¼oz flaked almonds, toasted

Method

Spoon the yoghurt into two glasses, top with half the berries, and then repeat the layers.

Sprinkle with the flaked almonds and serve.

Garlic mushroom frittata

Preparation time less than 30 mins

Cooking time 10 to 30 mins

Ingredients

low-calorie cooking spray

250g/9oz chestnut mushrooms, sliced

1 small garlic clove, crushed

1 tbsp thinly sliced fresh chives

4 large free-range eggs, beaten

freshly ground black pepper

For the salad

1 Little Gem lettuce, leaves separated

100g/3½oz cherry tomatoes, halved

1/3 cucumber, cut into chunks

Method

Spray a small, flame-proof frying pan with oil and place over a high heat. (The base of the pan shouldn't be wider than about 18cm/7in.) Stir-fry the mushrooms in three batches for 2-3 minutes, or until softened and lightly browned. Tip the cooked mushrooms into a sieve over a bowl to catch any juices – you don't want the mushrooms to become soggy.

Return all the mushrooms to the pan and stir in the garlic and chives, and a pinch of ground black pepper. Cook for a further minute, then reduce the heat to low.

Preheat the grill to its hottest setting. Pour the eggs over the mushrooms. Cook for five minutes, or until almost set.

Place the pan under the grill for 3-4 minutes, or until set.

Combine the salad ingredients in a bowl.

Remove from the grill and loosen the sides of the frittata with a round-bladed knife.Turn out onto a board and cut into wedges. Serve hot or cold with the salad.

Extra-lean burger and salad

Preparation time less than 30 mins

Cooking time 10 to 30 mins

Ingredients

low-calorie cooking spray

½ small onion, finely chopped

100g/3½oz Portobello mushrooms, finely chopped

250g/9oz extra-lean beef mince (under 5% fat)

2 tsp finely chopped fresh thyme (or ½ tsp dried thyme)

freshly ground black pepper

For the salad

1 Little Gem lettuce, leaves separated

120g/4½oz cherry tomatoes, sliced

1/3 cucumber, sliced

Method

Spray a small frying pan with oil and cook the onion and mushrooms over a medium heat for five minutes, or until well softened, stirring regularly. Tip into a heatproof bowl and leave to cool for five minutes.

Add the beef, thyme and lots of ground black pepper. Mix well and form into two balls. Flatten into burger shapes, each around 2cm/¾in thick.

Clean the pan and return to the hob. Spray with a little more oil and cook the burgers over a medium-low heat for 10 minutes, turning occasionally, until browned on the outside and cooked through inside.

Serve the burgers with lettuce, tomatoes and cucumber.

Chicken and sweetcorn soup

Preparation time less than 30 mins

Cooking time 10 to 30 mins

Ingredients

1½ chicken stock cubes

198g tin sweetcorn, drained

100g/3½oz skinless cooked chicken meat, cut into small pieces

25g/1oz cornflour

6 spring onions, trimmed and finely sliced

1 large free-range egg, well beaten

freshly ground black pepper

freshly chopped parsley, to garnish (optional)

Method

Put the stock cubes in a large saucepan and pour in 900ml/1⅔ pints water. Bring to the boil, stirring occasionally to dissolve the stock cubes. Add the sweetcorn and chicken and simmer gently for 3 minutes, stirring regularly.

Mix the cornflour with 3 tablespoons cold water in a small bowl. Stir the spring onions and the cornflour mixture into the stock and cook, stirring constantly, for 3–4 minutes, or until thickened. Season to taste with pepper. Remove the pan from the heat.

Pour the beaten egg over the hot soup and very lightly stir with a fork to distribute the egg strands. Ladle the soup into warmed bowls and scatter with parsley, if using.

Adaptable bean soup

Preparation time less than 30 mins

Cooking time 10 to 30 mins

Ingredients

2 onions

2 carrots

2 tbsp olive oil, plus extra for drizzling

3-4 ripe tomatoes

1 bay leaf

a few large handfuls of pre-cooked cannellini beans

vegetable stock

a few slices of orange peel

1 parmesan rind, or vegetarian alternative, optional

salt and freshly ground black pepper

1 handful chard stalks (and leaves if young)

fresh parsley, chopped

French stick, to serve

Method

Roughly chop the onions and carrots Warm a little olive oil in a large pan on a low heat and add the onions and carrots. Chop the tomatoes and add them to the pan with a bay leaf. Add the cannellini beans, followed by the vegetable stock - enough to cover. I like to add a couple of bits of orange peel at this stage, followed by the parmesan rind.

Season generously with salt and freshly ground black pepper and let the soup bubble. Chop the chard stalks and add to the liquid. (You could use any other greens you like.) Add plenty of chopped parsley, then add the chard leaves. Serve with some toasted French stick or ciabatta and a drizzle of olive oil.

Chapter 10: How Does A Water Fast Work?

Water speedy is while someone only drinks water and refrains from consuming.

There is not any unique quantity of time that water speedy need to final, even though in keeping with clinical tips, simply the maximum amount of time is normally among 24 hours and three days.

People have fasted for non secular or spiritual competencies all through records. But within the herbal fitness and nicely being moves, water fasting is now not unusual, regularly together with meditation. A form of rapid within the path of which you are exceptional allowed to drink water is referred to as water fast.

Water fasts normally last 24–seventy hours. Without scientific guidance, you shouldn't maintain to water rapid for delivered than this era of time.

People test with water fasting for the subsequent reasons:

For a non secular or religious cause

To reduce body fat

To "detox."

For health reasons

Getting equipped for a surgical procedure

The number one motivation for water fasting is to decorate one's health.

In reality, severa research have associated water fasting with a number of high-quality health benefits, together with a reduced threat of diabetes, coronary coronary heart disease, and some sorts of most cancers.

Water speedy also can inspire autophagy, a way thru which your body gets rid of and recycles damaged, old additives of your cells.

A form of rapid sooner or later of which you are only familiar to drink water is referred to as water speedy. It has various dangers but is associated with a reduced chance of persistent contamination and autophagy.

The water fast serves as the premise for popular diets similar to the lemon detox cleanse. You are best accredited to consume a concoction of lemon juice, water, maple syrup, and cayenne pepper more than one instances every day for as masses as 7 days in a few unspecified time in the future of the lemon detox cleanse.

In a scientific putting, sufferers have mechanically located for symptoms and signs of distress including a horrible flavor in the mouth, lower decrease again pain, pores and pores and skin rashes, mucous membrane discharges, headaches, irritability, nausea, or vomiting. Additionally, everyday urine and blood tests are finished.

Many people who exercise water fasts at home accomplish that with out expert help or the safety of medical tracking. People may observe pointers posted online or in periodicals due to the truth the device is quite clean.

Water fasting is easy, but that doesn't make it smooth or strong. You are nice commonplace to take water inside the direction of fasting. Typically, you eat 2 to three liters of water each day (ideally, water intake is probably at the higher prevent of that variety because of the fact you'll now not get the water you generally get from meals).

Water fasting is volatile and may be lethal if practiced for an prolonged period of time.

Preparing for a Water Fast

How to begin a water speedy is not problem to any medical pointers. However, positive populations should now not speedy without a physician's supervision.

People with gout, diabetes (which include sorts 1 and a couple of), consuming problems, aged people, pregnant girls, and kids are covered on this elegance.

Expect to experience exhausted and occasional on electricity in the course of a fast because of the truth the frame isn't always getting the nourishment it wishes.

People who're hungry can also revel in inclined, woozy, or dizzy, and if those signs are extreme, it is critical to consume a few element.

Energy conservation techniques consist of having hundreds of rest, sitting down, and keeping off strenuous hobby. It isn't uncommon to enjoy grouchy or exhausted after now not eating. If a person starts offevolved to experience lost or pressured at the same time as fasting, they need to touch a clinical scientific doctor.

It's a first-rate concept to spend 3–four days getting your body organized for a fast if you have in no way performed one earlier than.

By eating smaller portions at every meal or fasting for a part of the day, you could attain this.

Water Swift (24–seventy hours)

You aren't accepted to devour any food or liquids in some unspecified time in the future of a water rapid.

Typically, during a water rapid, humans consume to three liters of water day by day. A 24-72 hour water speedy is not unusual.

Lengthier water fasts without scientific supervision aren't recommended because of potential health risks.

In order to avoid moving into an twist of fate, a few oldsters which can be fasting on water can also feel vulnerable or dizzy and can want to chorus from working heavy machine or running a car.

Post-fast (1–three days)

You have to repress the preference to eat a heavy meal after the water speedy.

This is in reality so uncomfortable symptoms and signs and symptoms and signs and symptoms may not be introduced on with the useful resource of a heavy meal following a short.

Take a smoothie or smaller meals to break your rapid rather. As you get greater comfortable, you may begin to introduce massive food periodically at some stage inside the day.

Particularly important following extended fasts is the put up-speedy duration.

This is because of the opportunity that you may growth refeeding syndrome, a situation that may be deadly and causes rapid changes in the frame's fluid and electrolyte balances.

The common period of this phase is in the end, but the ones who've fasted for three or extra days may additionally furthermore need up to 3 days earlier than they feel prepared to consume massive food.

A post-fast phase generally lasts among 24 and seventy hours after the water rapid. If you are new to water fasting, you can choice to spend three–four days getting your frame organized with the aid of ingesting an awful lot tons less or going without meals for a part of the day.

Chapter 11: Potential Advantages Of A Water Fast

Studies on every human beings and animals have associated water fasting to some of health blessings. Short-time period fasting is probably effective for people who have precise issues as risk elements. Among them are:

Heart disorder

High ldl cholesterol and blood strain

Having diabetes and being overweight

These risks are frequently related. The frame will use fats as an opportunity energy supply if it can't get entry to carbs, which can be its primary gas deliver. Therefore, a quick might also additionally moreover purpose weight reduction due to the fact the frame burns down stored fats to provide strength.

The Academy of Nutrition and Dietetics states that a nutritious weight-reduction plan mixed with ordinary workout is the terrific method to little by little dropping weight.

Additionally, it's essential to make the effort to modify a few dietary practices, which include reducing again on the intake of sugary substances and snacks.

Additional advantages of water fasting for health consist of;

1. Autophagy can be Encouraged.

Old additives of your cells get broken down and recycled through a gadget referred to as autophagy.

Numerous studies on animals suggests that autophagy could probably offer a few form of defense in competition to situations collectively with most cancers, Alzheimer's, and coronary heart disorder.

For example, autophagy can also stop the accumulation of damaged mobile additives, that is a chance trouble for numerous malignancies. By doing this, cancerous cells won't be able to make bigger.

Water fasting appears to enhance autophagy, in keeping with animal studies. Autophagy also can moreover beneficial useful resource in extending existence, steady with animal research.

Nevertheless, studies on disease prevention, autophagy, and water fasting is scarce in human topics. Before suggesting it to stimulate autophagy, more research is needed.

2. Potential Blood Pressure Reduction

Longer water fasts beneath a doctor's supervision had been tested to have a blood stress-reducing impact on human beings with high blood pressure.

A water fasts for an average of 17 days even as being below medical institution remedy changed into validated to lower systolic blood strain in a check of forty eight obese or overweight humans.

Additionally, LDL (awful) cholesterol and inflammatory levels were verified to have advanced.

In a similar vein, a completely unique take a look at decided that water fasting may need to substantially lower blood strain stages and body weight in those with immoderate blood stress.

The relationship among brief-term water fasts (amongst 24 and seventy two hours) and blood pressure however desires to be studied very well.

three. Potentially makes Leptin and Insulin extra Sensitive

Important hormones which have an impact on the body's metabolism encompass insulin and leptin. Leptin makes the body experience whole, at the same time as insulin aids within the storage of vitamins from the bloodstream.

According to research, water fasting can also growth your frame's sensitivity to leptin and insulin. These hormones artwork better even as the frame is extra sensitive.

For example, having greater insulin sensitivity makes your body extra powerful in decreasing blood sugar levels. Being extra leptin sensitive, but, may additionally permit your body to cope with starvation cues greater correctly, for that reason reducing the chance of becoming overweight.

4. It May Reduce the Risk of a Number of Chronic Illnesses.

Water fasting can also help reduce the danger factors for continual illnesses like diabetes, most cancers, and coronary heart sickness, regular with a few studies. Thirty wholesome adults fasted on water for twenty-four hours as a part of a have a look at. They had extensively decreased blood triglyceride stages after the quick, that's a threat thing for coronary coronary heart illness.

Additionally, a few look at shows that water speedy might also moreover moreover protect the coronary heart from the damage because of free radicals.

Free radicals are unsteady molecules that may damage some mobile additives. They are identified to be worried in a number of persistent problems.

Additionally, investigations on humans and animals have placed that fasting on water can also moreover inhibit the genes that sell the increase of cancer cells. It may additionally furthermore decorate the consequences of chemotherapy.

Remember that little studies has tested the consequences of water fasting in people. Before making suggestions, more human topics want to be studied. According to analyze, fasting on the water can boom autophagy and decrease the hazard of a number of chronic ailments. However, animal or short-time period research makes up the bulk of studies. Before suggesting it, more studies is wanted.

Chapter 12: Water Fasting Dangers And Risks

Water fasting consists of fitness dangers even though it may probably offer wonderful benefits.

Here are severa dangers and dangers related to water fasting.

1. Could Lose the Incorrect Kind of Weight

Water fasting limits power, so that you'll likely shed pounds quick.

Unfortunately, you can lose lots of weight inside the beginning from water, carbohydrates, and likely even a bit little bit of muscle tissue.

2. Possible Dehydration

Water speedy might also moreover bring about dehydration, regardless of the weird-sounding notion.

This is due to the fact that amongst 20 and 30 percent of the water you consume every day comes from food.

You might not be receiving enough water if you're consuming the identical amount of water however not eating food.

Dizziness, nausea, headaches, constipation, low blood strain, and reduced productiveness are all signs and symptoms of dehydration. You may additionally want to drink more than normal to save you dehydration.

3. Orthostatic Hypotension would probable arise.

Orthostatic hypotension can result from dehydration delivered on via water fasting. When you rise up, your blood pressure drops, that may motive you to sense lightheaded, dizzy, or maybe faint.

You may additionally need to keep away from riding or the use of heavy device when you have orthostatic hypotension at the same time as fasting. Accidents can also need to rise up because of dizziness and the fainting danger. This type of fasting won't be the best choice for you if you go through these signs whilst on a water speedy.

4. Constipation: Eating food another time, particularly in extra portions, might also want to make you revel in ill and disappointed your belly after decreasing energy for a long time.

five. Potential for Refeeding Syndrome: Refeeding syndrome, a potentially lethal infection that entails rapid metabolic changes and commonly impacts patients who're critically malnourished, is much more likely to rise up in ladies and men who reintroduce meals too early after an prolonged fast. People with eating problems are much more likely to take refeeding syndrome into interest. To prevent refeeding syndrome in therapeutic settings, some guidelines endorse reintroducing calories very often (the use of dietary dietary supplements and growing by means of fine 10 to 30 energy steady with day).

6. May bring about Nutrient Shortages: Any fasting routine can boom your hazard of nutrient deficiencies.

Your body wishes certain vitamins, minerals, fatty acids, amino acids, and electrolytes to characteristic properly, all of that are restricted at the same time as you limit your caloric intake.

7. Unsafe Changes in Blood Pressure: If you devour too much water, hypotension may also additionally get up. Hypertension, or excessive blood strain, is the opportunity of hypotension, this is abnormally low blood pressure. Orthostatic hypotension, or abrupt dips in blood stress after repute up, is each unique possibility. The symptoms of orthostatic hypotension include lightheadedness and vertigo.

8. Hyponatremia: Also called water intoxication, hyponatremia takes area on the equal time as handiest water is used to top off the salt that is misplaced via sweating. Exercise shouldn't be completed even as on a water rapid due to the fact consuming food or eating sports activities activities activities beverages may not top off the salt you lose via perspiration.

nine. Unable to be Physically Active: This weight loss plan makes it difficult to be bodily lively, a crucial a part of health, similarly to the dangers of hyponatremia.

According to sure studies, fasting outcomes in decrease normal overall performance in plenty of health-related sports activities. Water fasting may also need to make a few scientific problems worse.

Despite the fast length of the water rapid, there are various conditions that it could make worse.

Without first getting guidance from a systematic professional, human beings with the subsequent clinical troubles should not water fast:

Gout: Water fasting also can moreover growth the synthesis of uric acid, a threat thing for gout assaults.

Diabetes: Both kind 1 and type 2 diabetics can also revel in an improved threat of horrible facet effects from water fasting. Chronic kidney ailment: Water fasting might also furthermore worsen kidney impairment.

Without any food to digest, your body may keep to offer extra belly acid than normal, inflicting heartburn. Eating Disorders: There is evidence that fasting may additionally stimulate disordered consuming patterns in a few people.

Water fasting consists of a number of risks and dangers, regardless of the reality that it might offer first-rate fitness blessings. For example, water fasting may additionally boom your threat for health problems like dehydration, blood stress fluctuations, and muscle loss.

10. Nutrient Deficiency

Your metabolism changes into a "fasting kingdom" even as you deprive your frame of nutrients, which is now and again called a "scenario earlier than the famine." When this takes area, your body turns to its reserves of protein and fat because it realizes it isn't getting what it desires. When you fast on water, you deny your body vitamins. Water fasting can rapid turn deadly, even within the 24-seventy hour range. Long-time period malnutrition can motive moderate symptoms like exhaustion, infection, anxiety, a reduction in blood stress, coronary heart rhythms, confusion, seizures, or perhaps lack of recognition.

Your frame is attempting to provide you with a warning that it's far miserable as it lacks the requirements for normal operation.

Chapter 13: Will A Water Fast Help You Lose Weight?

Water fasting, like specific types of fasting, can resource in weight loss There are exquisite fitness risks, despite the fact that. Intermittent fasting and change-day fasting are likely more a success strategies than water fasting for twenty-4-seventy two hours if you need to enjoy the advantages of fasting and decrease weight on the equal time.

These fasts provide similar fitness benefits however can be maintained for appreciably longer lengths of time thinking about they allow eating, lowering the opportunity of nutrient shortages. Even on the identical time as a water rapid can beneficial resource in weight loss, there are one of a kind fasting strategies which may be extra stable and but permit for weight reduction.

Those Who Should Not Fast

Not each person need to engage in water fasting. Older adults, human beings under 18, and people who've ingesting problems, are underweight, are pregnant or nursing, have coronary coronary heart situations, have kind 1 diabetes, have out of manage migraines, are receiving a blood transfusion, or are taking particular drug remedies should now not fast or have to are trying to find recommendation from a medical doctor in advance than doing so.

Safety

Water fast may not be suitable for absolutely everyone. Thus, it is also really beneficial to get scientific advice earlier than beginning one. Fasting may additionally have advantageous fitness benefits, however there are also vast troubles, especially if it's miles completed for an prolonged time period or with the useful aid of someone whose fitness or age makes them prone to bodily damage.

A person need to seek recommendation from a medical professional and preserve in thoughts fasting below supervision in the event that they have health troubles or intend to fast for a term more than 24 hours.

Water fasting isn't always safe for everybody and isn't encouraged for each person above the age of 18, human beings under the load restriction, or people who are underweight.

Tips

When now not going for walks or feeling well is the proper time to take a look at water fast. A person need to preferably rapid at the equal time as sound asleep in the comfort of their domestic. If someone has in no way fasted before, they'll maintain in mind starting with a one-day fast to test it out and make sure there are not any terrible outcomes. Only after consulting a systematic expert ought to you strive a fast lasting more than 3 days.

Fasting can be mentally and bodily draining, so humans need to carefully put together themselves through manner of

Eating well earlier than the quick

With materials which is probably high in electricity

Choosing a time on the manner to permit for rest, possibly on a day whilst they may be off from paintings

Avoiding fasting if they may be sick or extraordinarily exhausted

Avoiding annoying exercising

Possibly building up to a fast regularly, likely by using decreasing the scale of food.

It is crucial to eat suited sufficient water at some stage in the quick and space it out over the path of the day. When it is able to be tempting to eat greater beverages than regular whilst fasting, this have to be prevented. A individual need to no longer consume too much proper now after breaking a water rapid; as an opportunity, they should boom their intake grade by grade to save you nausea and stomach aches.

www.ingramcontent.com/pod-product-compliance
Lightning Source LLC
La Vergne TN
LVHW050817061126
851857LV00012B/856
9781738641253